DR. CAROLYN DEAN'S

Complementary
Natural Prescriptions
for Common Ailments

Keats Books of Related Interest

DR. CAROLYN DEAN'S

Complementary Natural Prescriptions for Common Ailments

by Carolyn Dean, M.D.

KEATS PUBLISHING, INC.

NEW CANAAN, CONNECTICUT

Dr. Carolyn Dean's Complementary Natural Prescriptions for Common Ailments is not intended as medical advice. Its intent is solely informational and educational. Please consult a health professional should the need for one be indicated.

DR. CAROLYN DEAN'S COMPLEMENTARY NATURAL
PRESCRIPTIONS FOR COMMON AILMENTS

Library of Congress Cataloging-in-Publication Data

Dean, Carolyn.
  [Complementary natural remedies for common ailments]
  Dr. Carolyn Dean's complementary natural remedies for common ailments / by Carolyn Dean.
      p. cm.
  Includes bibliographical references and index.
  ISBN 0-87983-632-6 : $12.95
  1. Naturopathy. 2. Homeopathy. I. Title. II. Title: Doctor Carolyn Dean's complementary natural remedies for common ailments.
RZ440.D43 1994
615.5'35—dc20   94-7751
                                                                      CIP

Printed in the United States of America

Published by Keats Publishing, Inc.
27 Pine Street (Box 876)
New Canaan, Connecticut 06840-0876

To Mom and Dad

Thanks for the healthy dose of common sense along with the cod liver oil.

CONTENTS

REMEDIES

INTRODUCTION

When You Can't Reach the Doctor

~ The information in this book is best used by patients once they have obtained a diagnosis from their doctor; it gives advice that has been compiled and utilized over the past eleven years in my practice and gives patients information and guidelines on taking responsibility for their bodies and on non-invasive treatments that can be used. This book and the enclosed treatment protocols may be used up to the point of needing drug or other medical therapy or while a person is waiting for results of investigations of his or her condition. In that interim, between discovering symptoms and clarifying a specific diagnosis, usually patients are not offered medical treatment. This period of time can be better utilized if patients investigate the natural remedies that can be used for their symptoms and begin natural therapy treatment.

Remember, conventional medicine and natural medicine are not mutually exclusive. It is no longer an either/or; it is both/and. Yes, you can have your cake and eat it too. All the benefits of highly sophisticated medical technology to diagnose disease and then the use of natural medicine, until you need surgery or stronger medication, gives you the best of both worlds. Sometimes the use of natural remedies solves the problem entirely. Sometimes it can speed healing and moderate the side effects of more conventional and invasive therapies.

The book is written in narrative form. A wide variety of conditions are discussed with treatment suggestions and at the end of the book a list of homeopathic remedies and tinctures are described. Often remedies described in the treatment section are discussed under the remedy section with more information to aid prescribing. Please study the remedies so that when a condition arises you will know which one is suitable to use for treatment.

This manual is not meant to take the place of good, sound medical advice and necessary treatment. If you have any questions at all be sure to consult with your medical doctor before using any of the following suggestions. In short, use your common sense and do not take any chances with your health. The actual dosages listed for various supplements and remedies are meant as a guideline. Again check with your doctor to decide your particular needs.

It is my heartfelt hope that the energy put forth and expressed in this book will enlighten and heal.

Carolyn Dean

DR. CAROLYN DEAN'S

*Complementary
Natural Prescriptions
for Common Ailments*

SYMPTOMS AND AILMENTS

Acne

❧ Acne can have either dietary or hormonal causes, due to the birth control pill or when it occurs premenstrually. The best advice is to avoid foods that may stimulate the secretion of oils on the skin of the face. These oils then plug the pores allowing the bacteria that live on our skin to infect the plugged pores and create the blemishes. For some people, simply avoiding sugar, chocolate and refined foods can change the picture. Other people have to avoid greasy foods such as fried foods and cut back on meat consumption, especially beef and pork.

In some cases, when blemishes occur on the back and buttocks as well as on the face, there can be an allergy. These blemishes are of a cystic type. In this case, milk should be discontinued. All dairy foods should be avoided for a period of three to four weeks to see if there is clearing of the acne. Various foods can be avoided for two to three weeks, then challenged one at a time for a two-day period to investigate whether these foods are indeed causing the problem.

Skin care is extremely important with acne. If the bacteria are removed from the skin twice a day and the pores are cleared of oil twice a day another cause of the condition is often eliminated. A good natural skin cleanser and facial mask such as clay

I

can be used on a regular basis. When beginning this treatment, sometimes the acne will appear to get worse as the underlying pores are being cleaned and debris comes to the surface. Oil-based makeup creates acne by blocking pores.

In some cases, a condition of acne with dry skin can occur. In these cases too much washing can increase the dryness. People with this problem need to take *cod liver oil*. Use 1 tablespoon per day and, in order to enhance absorption of natural oils and fats from food, do not drink water with your meals. See the chapter on **Dry Skin** for more information.

The following supplements appear to help most with acne. *Zinc* is important for wound healing. Begin with 25 to 50 mgs, three times a day for one month, then decrease to 25 mg a day. If you continue high levels of zinc above 25 mg, you can suppress copper. In this case, a hair analysis is sometimes helpful in determining mineral levels. *Vitamin E* (400 I.U.), *evening primrose oil, Efamol* or *gamma-linolenic oil* (3–4 capsules a day) and *vitamin A* (10,000–20,000 I.U.) per day are all useful oils for the health of skin, hair and nails.

Internal cleansing is an important factor with regard to acne. The body detoxifies any chemicals or excess toxins through the liver and the end products of this detoxification are eliminated through the intestines, the kidneys and the skin. If the kidneys and intestines are overloaded with toxins, then skin conditions can develop as too many waste products are being eliminated. Therefore, general cleansing can help the skin condition. The simplest form of cleansing is to increase the intake of fresh pure water and fiber.

If the bowel movements can be increased from one to two per day, we are sure that excess toxins are being released. Other gentle forms of cleansing include the intake of *aloe vera gel* which can be taken in juice once a day and *psyllium seed* taken as a bulking agent. However, acidophilus bacteria should be replaced if psyllium is used for more than one month at a time. Psyllium is taken either as a powder or capsule. The powder is shaken in a jar of water and followed by a second glass of pure water so that the bulking agent will not cause constipation instead of the expected cleansing action. Psyllium can be used for people with irritable bowel syndrome because it bulks up stools that are too loose or too solid. *Acidophilus* is taken as powder or capsules two doses per day or as plain yogurt. Acidophilus is the good bacteria of the intestines. (See the chapter on **Detoxification.**)

The homeopathic treatments that have been useful for acne are: *Hepar sulph.* 6c for painful acne that resembles tiny boils. *Graphites* 6c and *Antimonium tart.* 6c are used for acne that scars. There are many other homeopathic acne remedies but this treatment may require a constitutional assessment by a homeopathic physician for the full picture.

Above all, in the treatment of acne, it is important to realize that the use of oral antibiotics should be avoided where at all possible because the side effects of antibiotics can cause more problems than the acne itself. Oral antibiotics supposedly will kill the bacteria that create the facial blemishes but they also kill all intestinal bacteria, creating an extreme imbalance in the intestinal flora which can lead to the overgrowth of yeast or Candida in the intestines. (See the chapter on **Candidiasis.**) Candida overgrows when you are on the birth control pill and before your menstrual period. These hormones encourage yeast growth. Staphylococci bacteria on the skin plus Candida create boil-like acne blemishes. Treatment of Candida often decreases acne outbreaks.

Addictions

The treatment of addictions encompasses diet, remedies and behavioral and psychological counselling. I will give some of the remedies that can be useful in this process.

Coffee

The first advice would be to switch to black tea and take *Chamomilla* 30c, a homeopathic remedy for withdrawal symptoms of irritability, sensitivity and headaches. The dosage would be 4 drops orally three or four times a day but should not exceed six days in duration. Then black tea is stopped and *Chamomilla* can be continued for another few days. Then switch to herbal teas or a grain coffee, available in health food stores.

Smoking

For this addiction the remedies are:

Caladium, Nicotine and *Tabac* all homeopathics in the 6x or 6c potency, taken 4 drops three to six times a day.

The herbal tinctures *lobelia* or *Avena sativa*, taken 5 to 10 drops in four ounces of water three times a day.

A remedy called *Calc. phos.* can be used in the 6c potency for residual bronchitis that can remain after giving up cigarettes.

Also *fenugreek seed* tea, 1 teaspoon per cup of boiling water steeped for seven minutes, can help loosen the mucus that accompanies cigarette withdrawal.

The first month or so after quitting is often a difficult time because the small hair cells that line the bronchial tracts, beginning to grow again after being paralyzed for so long, start creating and clearing a lot of mucus. Although uncomfortable, this is a good sign.

Ear acupuncture can help to curb the craving for nicotine and to calm the irritability that usually ensues.

The other basic advice would be to maintain a good diet avoiding red meat, sugar, coffee and refined foods, taking a good multiple vitamin and mineral as well as zinc. *Zinc* at 30 to 50 mg a day will help bring back the taste buds so that food may be enjoyed more fully. Try to avoid switching one addiction for another. Most people who give up smoking begin eating sweets and gaining weight. Try to get to the bottom of the reason for the addiction and avoid being dependent on any substance.

Alcohol

Addiction to alcohol can be treated with homeopathic *Sulfuric acid* 6c four drops every few hours. This remedy is completely safe and has none of the properties of the real sulfuric acid in this extremely dilute form. It acts like Antabuse, a medical drug which is used to create a feeling of nausea and illness if a person drinks while taking it.

A rare remedy called *Quercus alba* 6c can curb the desire for alcohol. *Nux vomica* can curb desire as well as treat a hangover. Again 4 drops every hour for a hangover and three to four times a day to prevent desire for alcohol.

High doses of *vitamin C* will help metabolize alcohol but should not be used so a person can drink more. High doses would mean 2–8 grams throughout the day.

Alcoholism, a psychological and physical addiction, has to be treated in a whole-person manner. An excellent diet of grains, vegetables, fish, chicken and fruit that avoids refined foods, sugar, coffee and tea will prevent a person from craving alcohol. Some people feel that low blood sugar can trigger addiction to sugar or alcohol.

Vitamin therapy would consist of the already mentioned high doses of *vitamin C*, high doses of *niacinamide, B3* (500 mg from two to eight times a day), *B6* (100 mg, three times a day) and a *B complex* (50 mg, two or three times a day). *Zinc* is also important (50 mg per day for a month and then reduce to 25 mg per day) and a good *multiple vitamin and mineral supplement*.

Consider investigating this condition by reading books on low blood sugar and reading the chapter in this book on **Hypoglycemia**. Food allergies in the nutritional field can be synonymous with addiction. Read the chapter on **Allergies** in this book. Some of the first investigations into Candida overgrowth were due to diagnosing symptoms of a "drunk" disease in people who had not consumed any alcohol but appeared to be drunk. This turned out to be an overgrowth of yeast in their intestines which led to a fermentation process with ingested sugars which in turn created aldehydes, an alcohol byproduct. Therefore, some people consuming even a small amount of alcohol will have maximum effects and side effects. This can be due to a co-existing condition of Candidiasis. It is important to treat the Candidiasis as well as the alcoholism. Read the chapter on **Candidiasis** in this book.

Agoraphobia

This condition produces anxieties upon leaving the home due to a morbid dread of open or public places. Symptoms can extend to many anxiety-provoking situations. A person in an extremely stressful situation who begins to panic may forever after link that type of stress with a feeling of panic. On a physical level, if the blood sugar drops suddenly while the person is under stress, the adrenal reaction that is produced to push up the blood sugar can cause a fight or flight reaction which has some components of a panic attack. Therefore, a person will unknowingly link this hypoglycemic reaction with the stress and the panic attack and is likely to recreate a panic attack under similar stress.

Therefore, the treatment of agoraphobia is multi-faceted. For information on how to avoid low blood sugar, read the chapter on **hypoglycemia** in this book. Also avoid caffeine, sugar and alcohol. Vitamin supplementation can help especially with the *B vitamins*. B12 injections from your doctor can be especially beneficial. A non-yeast B source is the best to avoid further complications with possible yeast allergy or stimulating the growth of yeast or Candida in the body.

The best treatment is with support and behavior modification. To modify your behavior:

1. Face the fear.
2. Hum or sing, which activates the right side of the brain and deactivates the left side of the brain which is worrying and escalating the fear.
3. Celebrate each small victory against your fears. These small steps add up.
4. Try to move; don't lie down or give in to the fear.
5. Don't let fear of fear control your life.

The homeopathic remedies for agoraphobia are *Aconite, Kali arsenicum* and *Arsenicum*. These can be taken in the 6c potency, four drops as needed.

Allergies

⤜ Entire books have been written about allergies. The inhaled allergies are looked upon by conventional medicine as the main form of allergic reaction. For example, hay fever, with its symptoms of itchy runny eyes, runny nose and cough occurs in certain specific seasons, predominantly spring and fall. Spring allergies are usually to grasses and pollens. The best treatment is prevention. In the very early spring or late winter (February or March) begin an oral intake of homeopathic *Grasses and Pollens*. The dosage is 6c, 4 drops two to three times a day. If these are taken one month before the onset of the season, there is a high probability that the symptoms will be diminished. Similarly, in July, to avoid ragweed allergies, homeopathic ragweed, also called *Ambrosia* 6c, along with *Mold* 6c is taken two or three times per day. These can also be continued during the season if there are still some symptoms.

Vitamin supplementation would be high doses of *vitamin C* (up to 2 grams every four hours) as a natural antihistamine.

Some people also use *pantothenic acid* (500 mg two to three times a day) to support the adrenal glands which produce the natural cortisones that fight allergies. Other helpful supplements: *evening primrose oil* (four capsules per day) to support the immune system; *vitamin E* (400 I.U. per day) as an antioxidant; *magnesium* (300–400 mg per day) as a natural tranquillizer; *pancreatic enzymes* and *hydrochloric acid* (1–2 tablets or capsules with each meal) to prevent incomplete food digestion which can potentiate food allergies and *selenium* (200 micrograms a day) as an antioxidant.

Also, during allergy season, it is helpful to cut back on mucus-producing foods such as sugar, dairy and wheat. By doing so, you cut down the irritation in your mouth and nasal membranes and you are therefore less susceptible to irritation from inhaled pollens etc. The only food allergies recognized by most medical allergists are eggs, peanuts, nuts, fish, shellfish and strawberries, those which create an immediate IgE reaction of hives, asthma, or severe swelling of the throat and face. These immediate reactions are easy to spot and most people have identified what foods they should avoid. Added to this list are MSG or bisulphites that are used in food preparation or to keep salad greens looking fresh. Some people can have life threatening reactions to these invisible substances.

Other food allergies, mediated by the IgG immunoglobulins, display delayed reaction. The identification of these allergies is very difficult. Blood tests to determine these allergies are available in many laboratories in the U.S.

Otherwise, a person must obtain a list of the most common food allergens and do a process of elimination and avoidance of each particular food group for a three to four week period. Then a person does a challenge test of eating that food several times in a 48-hour period and observing reactions. This can be very time consuming but provides very useful information. The book that describes this process is *Dr. Mandell's Five Day Food Allergy Relief System* by Marshall Mandell, M.D.

Allergies can cause reactions from runny nose and abdominal

pain to irritable bowel, bladder irritation, skin reactions and cerebral reactions. Some people have anxieties and depression that are purely the result of the foods they are ingesting. It is important to investigate whether any of your symptoms could be allergies and for you to do your best to avoid those foods that are causing a problem. Some people find they react to many different substances in their environment and the best treatment is to be armed with information about the environment and your own body and to eliminate as many of these substances as possible.

For inhalant allergies, the air must be kept dry and clean with air conditioners, air cleaners and dehumidifiers. Make sure mold doesn't grow in these appliances because mold spores cause considerable allergy symptoms in susceptible people. Mold in bathrooms and basements can be cleaned away with bleaches or trapped with zeolite-clay powder.

Dust and dust mites, tiny microscopic insects that feed off dust, are the most common inhaled allergen. Vacuuming your mattress, covering it with plastic, washing your pillow and bed clothes frequently and removing carpeting from your bedroom floor will help. Sometimes after a bad cold with nasal congestion, people can develop hayfever or dust allergies because their mucous membranes become very sensitive. Then special cleaning will have to be done. Cleaning itself can lead to a sneezing attack. Use a cotton face mask or have a non-allergic person do the cleaning.

Pets can also be a problem with their hair, fur, dander, skin oils and secretions. They should be isolated from sleeping and living areas and a thorough cleaning of the areas they do inhabit must be done frequently.

Amenorrhea

❧ This is the delay or absence of the menstrual period. Primary amenorrhea is diagnosed when the period does not occur at the usual age in young women. If the period has not occurred by age 15 or 16, investigations are advised. However, if the patient is under 100 pounds or an extremely active athlete, this may account for the lack of menstruation. If, after cycling has been established, the period stops for over one year, then it can be a result of stress, either emotional or physical (including another disease process), overwork, anemia, grief or disappointment. The clinical investigation would, of course, include tests for pregnancy or anemia.

The natural treatment with homeopathic remedies would be:

Calc. carb.   6c, 4 drops three times a day, for overwork and exhaustion.

Ferrum met.   6c, 4 drops three times a day, for anemia and resulting weakness. An oral iron supplement would also be taken.

Ignatia   6c, 4 drops three times a day, for grief, fear of failure or disappointments causing the amenorrhea.

Rhus tox.   6c for a suppression of periods in an overactive athlete. 4 drops three times a day.

Sepia   6c for amenorrhea due to the birth control pill, a miscarriage or an abortion, 4 drops three times a day.

These remedies should only be used for a maximum period of two to three months. If more advice is needed, consult a homeopathic physician.

Anemia

 Low levels of hemoglobin have to be thoroughly investigated to determine blood loss, blood destruction or lack of blood production. The nutritional causes of anemia can be low iron, low copper or low B12 and folic acid. These can be determined by blood tests and hair analysis. The treatment of nutritional causes for anemia is supplementation. The best supplement is a synergistic combination of all the nutrients that are used in the production of hemoglobin including *B complex, folic acid, iron, copper, vitamin C* and additional *B6*. As for diet, red meat, prune juice, legumes, spinach, and blackstrap molasses are good sources of iron.

During pregnancy, the excess strain on the mother's blood supply will lower the blood levels from the normal 12 to 16 grams of hemoglobin by 1 or 2 grams. The supplements most required during pregnancy for the hemoglobin are *iron* and *folic acid*. The best source is a *chelated iron*, not the ferrous form of iron. The ferrous form is given in 300 mg doses but only 7 percent of it is absorbed and often causes constipation and dark stools. The *chelated irons* are more readily absorbed up to 80 percent; therefore less is required and less constipation results.

Folic acid has to be taken during pregnancy for the hemoglobin and to prevent birth defects. This is only available in adequate amounts by prescription; 5 mg one or two times a day is necessary throughout the pregnancy. It would also appear from various studies that the more natural the supplement used, the better it is for the body. The body may not be able to use synthetic forms of supplements as readily as natural ones. Herbs such as *kelp, watercress* and *nettles* are very rich in blood building nutrients. All dark green leafy vegetables are also excellent sources of iron. Homeopathic *Ferrum phos.* and *Ferrum met.*, best in the cell salt 6x form, help the body's absorption and use of iron.

Angina Pectoris

࿇ This is a condition in which the blood vessels of the heart either go into spasm or are blocked. The symptom is crushing chest pain which occurs on exertion and should be thoroughly investigated by a medical doctor. The treatments vary from different drugs to increase the circulation or increase the width of the blood vessels to surgery which replaces the arteries of the heart. The natural treatment that can be used in conjunction with medication and exercise is primarily diet to lower cholesterol. An optimal cholesterol level is 180 or lower. Above this number, cholesterol can clog the arteries. Below this level blocked arteries are very rare. The Pritikin diet offers a very strict but effective cholesterol lowering approach. The latest book on this topic that scientifically proves that heart disease can be reversed through diet, meditation and exercise is *Dr. Dean Ornish's Guide to Reversing Heart Disease*. Ornish's diet is strictly vegetarian. Some people may feel they need some fish and free-range chicken as well.

An optimum diet will help achieve an optimum weight. Excess weight puts a strain on the heart because all the extra miles of capillaries that feed the extra tissue have to be pumped by the heart.

Exercise also helps with weight loss and as a natural stress reducer. Walking is probably the best form of exercise and if an angina attack starts to come, just stop and rest. As endurance builds and circulation improves, health will return.

Smoking, of course, is out. It decreases dramatically the oxygen level throughout the body and the heart has to work furiously to try to keep the body oxygenated.

Supplementation includes vitamins and minerals such as *vitamin C* (2 grams per day) as an antioxidant; *vitamin E* (400–800 units per day) as an antioxidant; *magnesium* (500 mg per day) for heart spasms and palpitations; *B Complex* (50 mg once or twice daily) to calm the nervous system; and a good *multiple vitamin and mineral*. (Read the chapter on **Atherosclerosis**.)

An herbal tincture that is useful for the heart is *hawthorne berry* which can be used 5 to 10 drops in four ounces of water three times a day. *Spigelia* as a herbal tincture can be used for severe chest pain but should not be used in place of prescribed medication. Both tinctures and medication can be used simultaneously but one should not take chances with a life-threatening situation by stubbornly using only natural remedies. *Avena sativa* tincture can help treat palpitations (5 to 10 drops three or four times a day). The most common cause of heart palpitation is coffee intake and that should be stopped.

Anorexia

ॐ This condition is very complex and requires treatment on both the physical and psychological levels. One very important nutrient is *zinc*; some people with zinc deficiency have poor wound healing, white spots on the nails, increased susceptibility to infections and lack of sense of taste and smell. To anorexics, this could mean that food, having no taste, begins to feel revolting or disgusting and food is avoided. In bulimia, people may eat more and more food in order to get some sense of taste, eating stronger or sweeter food or binging on foods just to be satisfied. The treatment could be started with *zinc* (50 mg chelated, daily for at least a month). A good *multiple vitamin and mineral* with *copper* should be added so that the copper in the body will not be suppressed by the high zinc intake. There are several homeopathic remedies that have been considered useful for anorexia; these should be administered by a qualified homeopathic physician. It is also very important to do a thorough medical workup and make an appointment with an Eating Disorder Clinic to investigate and treat all aspects of this condition.

Antibiotics

ॐ (See SINUS INFECTIONS)

Anxiety

᷑ Most of the recommendations for anxiety are found in this book under the heading **Agoraphobia**. One aspect of anxiety that is becoming more recognized is the effect of electricity on our nervous system. It is said that electricity is like the extension of our nervous system onto our skin which may make some sensitive people more aware or susceptible to the stresses of our society. The works of Marshall McLuhan can be studied in this regard.

Arteriosclerosis

᷑ Also known as hardening of the arteries, arteriosclerosis is commonly caused by elevated cholesterol. Cholesterol, necessary for many body functions such as creating hormones and protecting the nerves, can also, in excess amounts, build up in the arteries.

Research is now finding that cholesterol also acts as an antioxidant that sponges up excess free radicals that cause damage in the body. Therefore, the more free radicals, the higher the cholesterol goes to contain them. So one treatment might be to get rid of the free radicals, rather than the cholesterol.

However, arteries are in fact irritated or damaged by excess cholesterol. It sets up a reaction which also allows the build up of calcium, thus causing the hardening of the arteries. As time passes, this situation can cause narrowing of the arteries and symptoms leading to stroke, heart attack and blocked circulation to the extremities. The best treatment is prevention. The Pritikin diet, which lowers fat intake to 10 percent of calories, is the most effective for lowering cholesterol and helping to actually dissolve the plaque of cholesterol from the arteries. A combination of diet, regular exercise and supplements will help lower cholesterol levels. The main foods to avoid are sugar, fried foods, dairy and animal products that have high fat content. The strictness of the diet depends on the severity of the disease.

The supplements to use are *vitamin C*, which helps heal the artery damage at a dosage of 1,000–2,000 mg per day; *vitamin E*, which acts as a blood thinner, 400–800 I.U. per day; *bioflavins* as part of the *vitamin C complex*, 250–500 mg per day, which also help heal arteries; *calcium* and *magnesium* in a ratio of 1:1. Calcium helps lower blood pressure as does magnesium. It is interesting that the newest heart medicines are calcium channel blockers and actually the best calcium channel blocker is magnesium because calcium and magnesium work in unison. Calcium and magnesium are used together, 500 mg of calcium and 500 mg of magnesium, one to two a day. *Lecithin* capsules have an effect on balancing the cholesterol and bile in the liver. *Trace minerals* are also important in a good *multi-vitamin and mineral*.

Flaxseed oil (in a light-proof bottle) can be used on salads and hot cereal. This is a polyunsaturated oil rich in linoleic acid. The best oil for cooking is olive oil and the relatively new canola oil. These oils are monosaturates and won't get denatured on heating. Recent studies show that people who use olive oil have half the average rate of heart disease. Even though it is a fat, it actually causes the undesirable LDL cholesterol to fall and maintains the good HDL cholesterol. If one were to choose between butter and the specially made polyunsaturated margarines, butter is actually healthier. These manufactured margarines cause more harmful oxidative effects than the completely saturated butter. Read Udo Erasmus's book *Fats and Oils*; it is quite a revelation.

The Pritikin diet stresses fiber as well as vegetable protein including soy products. Dr. John Anderson's work on fiber and cholesterol has proven that two to three oat bran muffins and a serving of a bean or legume dish per day will lower cholesterol. Vegetarians have far fewer heart attacks and strokes and have lower cholesterol levels in general. Dr. Dean Ornish's work *Re-*

versing Heart Disease goes into diet as well as lifestyle and is the most comprehensive natural treatment for heart disease.

One important aspect of cholesterol metabolism is that it can be reabsorbed back into the system instead of leaving through the gut. This means detoxification and cleansing are very important to pull as much cholesterol out as possible. If there are too many colonies of abnormal bacteria in the colon, then the cholesterol will be reabsorbed by an intricate mechanism. Therefore, a high fiber diet, bulking agents such as *psyllium*, and detoxifying with *aloe vera gel* are all important. (See the chapter on **Detoxification**.)

Please refer to the discussion under **Angina** as well as the discussion under **Allergies** for more information. Exercise is also extremely important beginning with slow short walks and increasing gradually to allow the blood vessels to spread and multiply to increase the circulation in all parts of the body.

Arthritis

 This is a very complex and multi-faceted disease. The best resource book available on arthritis that gives many modalities for treatment is *Arthritis* by Jan DeVries.

Arthritis merely means inflammation of the joints. A diagnosis of arthritis is made by x-rays, blood tests and clinical examinations. If the x-rays and blood tests are essentially normal but the patient continues to experience swelling of the joints, stiffness and pain, then other causes must be investigated. Some people have joint symptoms due to food allergies, Candidiasis or post-viral infections such as Epstein-Barr or chronic mononucleosis. The arthritic symptoms are caused by antigens from foods and antibodies from the blood that join together in the blood and create antigen-antibody complexes which then can deposit in any area of the body. The joints are a frequent area of deposition and once in that area they may appear to be arthritic.

First, the individual should try an elimination diet of the most allergenic foods such as wheat, dairy, corn and sugar and determine if there is an improvement. Then, one might try to eliminate the most likely yeast-growing foods such as sugar, bread with yeast, moldy foods, cheeses and excess fruits and see if it changes the joint symptoms. A common cause of small-joint arthritis is allergy to the deadly nightshade family of potato, tomato, green pepper, tobacco, eggplant and paprika. These should be avoided for at least two months to determine possible allergy.

Reaching optimum weight is also very important because any excess weight on an inflamed joint creates more pain.

Women, at the time of menopause when their periods begin to disappear, often get arthritic symptoms. I wonder if the absence of the monthly period which served to rid the body of toxins, means that instead the toxins are building up in the joints. I therefore advise patients going through menopause to go on a detoxification program. (Please see the chapter on **Detoxification**.) Treatment for arthritis is a good healthy diet, including whole grains, vegetables, nuts, seeds, fruit, fish and chicken.

Simple advice for relief from the pain of arthritis includes:

1. Castor oil compresses or rubs. This oil has been proven to increase lymphatic blood flow to clear away toxins and inflammatory by-products.

2. Gentle stretches and exercise, tai chi and yoga are especially helpful. Hydrotherapy in a heated pool can do wonders. Do gentle exercise in the pool or swim. Massage therapy really helps the circulation and helps clear away inflammatory by-products.

3. Simple meditation, prayer or affirmations help to calm and remove stress. The Silva Method is a nonsectarian meditation-affirmation technique that has an excellent worldwide reputation.

4. Be careful with heating pads and ice. Use heat only on

stiff joints and for only a short time. Use ice if a joint is hot and inflamed. Be sure to check with your doctor for special instructions on your case.

Supplements that help arthritic symptoms are *vitamin C*, 1 gram three times a day along with *pancreatic enzymes*, 2 tablets three times a day. This in conjunction with vitamin C acts as an anti-inflammatory which has proven to be as effective as most anti-inflammatory medications. Also, high doses of the *B vitamins* have been helpful. Some people respond to *niacinamide*, 500 mg 2 to 6 tablets a day and *vitamin B6*, 100 mg 1–3 times a day. Some people also respond to *devil's claw*, an herb that often helps the symptoms of arthritis. Take 2–6 capsules per day.

Studies using *evening primrose oil*, *flaxseed oil*, and *fish oils* demonstrate improved joint mobility and decreased inflammation. They are natural anti-inflammatories.

There are many homeopathic remedies for arthritis but since it is a chronic condition it requires the skills of a homeopathic physician to take the case history and prescribe the best remedy. Read the chapters on **Allergies, Detoxification, Candidiasis, Epstein-Barr** and **Digestion** to understand your condition and in order to help yourself more.

Asthma

This is a condition of spasm of the bronchial tubes which results in shortness of breath and wheezing and can be life threatening. Asthma is more and more being recognized as both a stress and allergic reaction. This means a person can use medication and also natural methods to give more relief and to gradually decrease medications.

One very important suggestion is to participate regularly in relaxing exercises such as yoga, swimming or tai chi. Diet is extremely important. Some people have allergies to any number of inhaled or ingested substances which can trigger asthma attacks. Such substances can include MSG, salt, food additives or aspirin. It is felt that asthmatics do not digest their food because of a deficiency of hydrochloric acid in their stomach. Please see the chapter on **Digestion** for more information.

If you get asthma at night, be sure you have a dust-free bedroom. Remove the carpets, cover your mattress with plastic and wash pillows and bed covers frequently.

Also avoid smoke-filled environments, incense, cigarettes or wood-burning fires. Use air conditioners and air cleaners.

Vitamins that are useful include *vitamin C* (2,000 to 4,000 mg per day) as a natural antihistamine; *pantothenic acid* (500 mg, 2–6 per day) as adrenal support; non-yeast *B-complex* vitamins (50 mg, 1–2 per day). B6 is especially useful in treating asthma.

Homeopathic remedies for asthma include *Arsenicum* 6c especially for night asthma with panics, 4 drops every few minutes. If the attack does not subside, medical assistance should be sought. There are lists of suitable homeopathic remedies for asthma, which include *Aconite* and *Nux vomica*, that should be studied.

Herbal remedies such as *Brigham tea* have natural ephedra which is a bronchial relaxant but one would use no more than one to two cups a day. Acupuncture is also very helpful for asthma, especially ear acupuncture which can relax the lung point and diminish symptoms.

In an acute attack, take in lots of fluids so the lungs don't get dry and turn the mucus into dry plugs that block the breathing more. Use *fenugreek tea* to liquify mucus and inhale steam or use a humidifier. People in fact do not realize how much moisture can be lost during a fever or an asthma attack. So if you aren't urinating out as much as you are taking in, be aware that you are getting dehydrated.

Athlete's Foot

෴ Athlete's foot is a very common condition caused by a fungus which lives on the skin and nails of the foot. The best conditions for its growth are warm, dark and damp areas. People in tropical climates are more prone to this infection, but sweaty footgear is a common cause of this infection in North America. The skin, in the acute stage, can be blistered and cracked and discharging clear liquid. However, most often it is in a chronic stage of irritation and itchiness. In the acute stage, keep the area dry and uncovered; for the inflammation, soak the foot in various solutions, such as clay mixtures with one tablespoon of white zeolite clay or green clay; one tablespoon of salt; or one tablespoon of baking soda in a quart of water. *Taheebo tea* can be used also to soak the feet. This tea is made from the bark of a tree that grows in Brazil that won't allow fungi or mold to grow on its surface, therefore exhibiting powerful antifungal properties. A tablespoon of this bark boiled for an hour in a quart of water can be used over and over again. It merely has be to be reheated before reusing. After soaking, which lessens the inflammation, pain and itching, antifungal creams and lotions can be applied.

There are many over-the-counter medications which can be used two or three times a day but must be continued for at least four weeks. The preparations available in the health food stores include *tea tree oil*, which is a potent antifungal, and *garlic oil*, which is also a powerful antifungal oil. *Vitamin E oil* can be used because it encourages oxygen in an area which is trying to avoid oxygen because fungi grow best in an anaerobic environment. *Zeolite powder*, used for removing the odor from footwear, helps to trap fungus spores, to dry athlete's foot blisters and to keep the foot dry inside the shoes. Therefore, after soaking the feet, scrubbing them to remove any dead skin that can harbor the fungus, and drying the feet well—perhaps even with a hairdryer—the whole foot can be powdered with zeolite or clay powder. Then, put on fresh cotton socks and put another half teaspoon of powder directly inside your shoes. Change your socks several times a day if your feet perspire heavily, and change your shoes once or twice a day, because they hold the moisture and the fungus. These recommendations do not have to be as strict if the clay powder is absorbing the moisture and also helping to kill the fungus. The worst types of shoes and boots are rubber and plastic, which hold sweat and moisture inside.

People often ask me why they get athlete's foot while their next-door locker-mate has never been bothered. Some people of course are more susceptible, and if you are susceptible, prevention also dictates that you should cover your feet in areas where people are going barefoot, such as gyms, spas, swimming pools, etc. However, your susceptibility may not be just a stroke of bad luck, but may be due to an overgrowth of yeast on your mucous membranes and skin, which would then make you more susceptible to fungal growths. The yeast mainly grows in our gastrointestinal tract, but when it overgrows, it can cause oral thrush in the mouth, vaginitis in women, and it can grow on the skin and not even be detectable but create an environment for other fungi to grow. Treatment of this condition includes avoiding sugar, bread with yeast, dairy, and alcohol for a period of time to see if the yeast can be starved in the gastrointestinal tract. See the chapter on **Candidiasis**, which fully explains this condition.

Baby Feeding

ᐲ This section is geared toward infant feeding to avoid allergies. If the mother has allergies or sensitivities to specific foods, then the child has a good chance of being allergic. Even while nursing, the baby may experience gas or colic and this may be treated by eliminating certain foods from the mother's diet.

These foods, or overuse of these foods may cause a problem: nuts, milk, cheese, wheat, corn, chocolate, fish or—on an individual basis—just about any food can be the culprit.

In general, try to rotate foods as much as possible. Because we eat the same foods day after day we are likely causing food sensitivities.

Infant Feeding Guide

The First Six Months

Offer only:
Breast milk
Commercial modified cow's milk formula
Commercial soy bean formula
Water
Supplemental vitamin A and D from cod liver oil, and vitamin
  C, from three months.

Six to Twelve Months

Breast milk or the chosen formula
Water between feedings
Solid foods are introduced one at a time starting with vegetables. Three meals a day are usual by nine to twelve months.
  Yogurt or kefir from nine months.

VEGETABLES (COOKED)
  Begin with: peas, squash, carrots, green beans, red beets, sweet potatoes. Add later: potato, broccoli, cabbage, dried peas and beans, vegetable combinations, celery, asparagus. Watch for a reaction if the infant is on a formula and begins peas, green beans, fresh or dried or any vegetable combination. There can be a cross reactivity between these foods.

FRUITS (COOKED)
Begin with: apple, peach, banana. Add later: apricots, plums, pears, pineapple, cherries, grapes.

MEATS AND DAIRY
Begin with: beef, pork, lamb (hormone and antibiotic free). Add later: fish (salmon, tuna, turbot), shellfish (shrimp, crab, oyster), fowl (turkey, chicken, duck), dairy (yogurt, cottage and soft cheese).

CEREALS
Begin with: rice, oats, rye. Add later: millet, barley, wheat and corn.

Food Feeding Rules

Always introduce one new food at a time.

Watch for colds or runny nose, cough, sneezing, increased fussiness, diarrhea, rash, and vomiting. Try to correlate with the foods eaten that day or the day before.

Rotate foods. A food should be given only every third day.

Use only water as a between-meal beverage.

Avoid until after one year old:
Orange, grapefruit, lemon, lime, eggs, ham, bacon.

Avoid until after two years old:
Peanut butter, chocolate, cola, candy, nuts, nut butters, spices (especially cinnamon), food colorings, artificial flavorings, whole milk, seed butters.

FOODS TO AVOID IN GENERAL
Artificial flavors and colors
Coffee and tea
Chocolate, cocoa, colas
Flavor enhancers (MSG, citric acid)
Preservatives (BHT, BHA, nitrites)
Refined starches, (cornstarch, white flour)
Sugar (brown, white, corn syrup, molasses)

FOODS TO LIMIT IN GENERAL
Honey and maple syrup

Natural sugars (dried fruits, grapes, plums)
Milk
Pasta (noodles, spaghetti, macaroni)

FOODS TO USE
Brown rice
Dried peas and beans
Fresh fruits
Fresh meats, fish, poultry (free-range, antibiotic- and
  hormone-free and grain-fed)
White whole milk, goat, or cottage cheese
Whole grain cereals
Whole grain flour
Water (from a purified source)

Baby Tips

◆1. Most babies thrive on demand feeding, not schedule feeding. Try to feed in a more vertical than horizontal position. This prevents milk from being sucked into the eustachian tubes and prevents ear infections. For cracked nipples, *vitamin E oil* from capsules is great and if the baby gets some during a feeding it is good for them, unlike most other creams or ointments. Proper nipple positioning into the baby's mouth prevents cracked nipples. Call your local LaLeche League for firsthand information and assistance with breast feeding.

◆2. Babies swallow a lot of air when feeding and really need to be burped.

◆3. Turn babies frequently; they can't turn over themselves. The best position to prevent SIDS (sudden infant death syndrome) is on the back.

◆4. Cavities often plague the children of health-conscious

parents. This stems from giving babies bottles with natural juices at bedtime. The extremely high fructose content drills holes in the teeth. Never use anything but water in a bottle if it is being used as a soother.

5. Constipation is often observed when switching from breast to bottle or when introducing solids. The formula may be too high in solutes and may need to be diluted. Or, it may be a reaction to processed dairy or wheat. Try avoiding these foods for two to three weeks to see if it makes a difference. Increase diluted fruit juices. Increase water feeding. Stress and tension in or between the parents can translate into a holding back by the child which can manifest as constipation.

6. For colic in breast-fed babies, especially if your baby burped or hiccoughed in the womb, watch what you eat. The baby may be reacting to something that doesn't agree with her or him in your diet. Cut out strong-tasting foods first; then cut out dairy and wheat. Read the chapter on **Colic**.

Pulsitilla for gentle, usually happy babies who need to be held, rocked and moved all the time. Use 6c, 4 drops in one tsp. of water several times a day as needed.

Chamomilla for whiny, irritated and irritating babies, who seem as frustrated as you feel. Use 6c, 4 drops in one tsp. of water several times a day.

7. Diarrhea is defined as more than four very loose, odorous, runny stools a day. Stop milk and dairy products and use water feedings for 24 hours. Make sure enough water is given to prevent dehydration. Then try normal feeding. If your baby is already drinking juices, use apple juice with ¼ tsp. carob powder in 4 oz. water.

8. For diaper rash, leave the diaper off for longer periods; *vitamin E ointment* or *zinc ointment* are very good. Talc or cornstarch are not necessary and can cause allergic reactions.

Some diaper rash may be due to an overgrowth of Candida or yeast. The yeast live in the bowel and the baby on passing through the birth canal can get a mouthful of yeast and be overgrown with this organism. If the baby has also had antibiotics early in life, this can contribute to the overgrowth. (Please read the chapter on **Candidiasis**.) The treatment for Candidiasis in babies is often to treat the breastfeeding mother and give the baby *acidophilus powder* and use *antifungal ointments* on the local irritation.

9. Fever in an infant is often quite frightening. A baby's temperature can rise very rapidly. It is important to have measures at hand to treat the fever and, if nothing seems to help, to be sure and go to a doctor or the emergency department for a diagnosis. Most often the fever is due to a viral infection, but it can be due to an ear infection, pneumonia or meningitis. A viral infection will run its course but the others often need an antibiotic. Dehydration can set in quite rapidly with infants. Be sure that your baby is producing urine. If not, dehydration is occurring and this alone can drive up the temperature.

To reduce a mild fever 99° to 102.5° F. (at 103° and higher, consult your doctor):

Vitamin C at 100 mg per hour crushed in water or juice (buffered C powder is good to have on hand). The only possible side effect is diarrhea.

Yarrow as an herb tea or in a bath. A lukewarm bath itself will help reduce the fever and aid hydration.

Belladonna 6c or 30c, 4 drops every 15 minutes. (Read the section on belladonna in the **Remedies** part of this book).

Aconite 6c or 30c, 4 drops every 15 minutes. (Read the section on aconite in the **Remedies** part of this book).

Ensure that the infant or child is not constipated; do whatever makes the stool soft—a gentle enema or suppository may be necessary. You may want to consult your doctor before attempting this measure.

Identify teething as a cause of fever.

If temperature rectally is 103.5° and the above therapies are not working, use *baby Tylenol* and call the doctor.

Dont's:

Don't use aspirin for babies; they can be allergic and it is linked to Reye's syndrome.

Don't use alcohol baths.

Don't panic.

10. Spitting up is quite common; it is not vomiting. It can be from eating too fast, when the parent is stressed while feeding the child, or food intolerance. Projectile vomiting should be investigated because it can mean a blockage to the food passing out of the stomach.

11. Teething. This stage of development is usually accompanied by fussiness, drooling and even slight fevers. For the irritability and crying, use *Chamomilla* 6c, 4 drops three times a day. For hot, sore gums, rub the powder from a crushed calcium tablet on the gums. For late teething, use homeopathic *Calc. carb.* 6c, 4 drops three times a day. The herbs *marshmallow root* and *licorice root* can be used to chew on and will help soothe the gums as well as help the teeth break through. Teething rings kept in the fridge can give a soothing coolness to hot gums.

Back Pain

 This can be a very frightening condition and could mean anything from a muscle spasm to an actual prolapsed or slipped disc. This occurs when the pad between each vertebrae is forced out from between the vertebrae and the bones are crushing or pressing the nerves that come off the spinal cord. The diagnosis definitely has to be clarified by a doctor. If the advice is bed rest, muscle relaxants and pain killers, a person can also use ice alternating with heat.

The following homeopathic remedies can be useful and are non-toxic.

Arnica 6c for pain, shock and swelling, 4 drops every half to one hour while pain is severe. If the pain is more like stiffness, *Rhus tox* 6c can be used in the same amounts. If there is definite nerve tingling and irritation, *Hypericum* 6c can be used.

The best treatment for pain in the acute injury period is ice. Never use heat on an acute inflammation. If the pain is chronic, use ice and heat (ten minutes of one, rest ten minutes and ten minutes of the other). You can use castor oil packs for both acute and chronic pain. Take an old hand towel and rub in four to five tablespoons of castor oil. Cover the affected area but ensure that your bed clothes are protected with plastic. You may use a heating pad on low to help the action but it works just fine at room temperature, too. Leave on at least one hour or overnight. Castor oil has been proven to reduce inflammation. Warm to moderately hot Epsom salts baths will help chronic back pain.

The nutrients for easing back pain are high doses of *vitamin C*, from 2–5 grams a day; *calcium* and *magnesium* in a one-to-one ratio 500 mg each 1–2 a day. Acupuncture is good for the treatment of back pain as are gentle and structured exercises. If a person is overweight, the excess strain of that weight on the back can aggravate the problem so a weight loss program is indicated for those people. Several recent studies have proven that the best care for acute and chronic back pain is by a good chiropractor. The best ones are those that work on the muscles as well as the bones and prescribe exercises. A good chiropractor teaches you how to take care of your own body rather than creating a dependency on him or her.

Prevention, of course, is the best treatment.

Learn how to lift by bending your knees and keeping your back straight. Don't twist your back to move an object; move your whole body.

A firm mattress that doesn't sag is very important. So is sleep position. Sleep on your back with support under your knees and under your head and neck. Or sleep on your side with support under your neck and head and another pillow between your knees. There are many styles of neck pillows available now. These have a rounded end which conforms to the shape of the neck, holding it in proper alignment during sleep. Chiropractors say that a person with a bad low back can have a corresponding problem in the neck and vice versa. Therefore, pay attention to the neck as well as the back.

Bad Breath

As with so many other conditions, I wonder if bad breath is just a symptom of a body out of balance. Most people think that bad breath comes from eating food that is highly spiced or very strong and just lingers in the mouth long after eating. These foods include the obvious ones such as garlic, onion, spicy and heavy meats and cheeses, fish, coffee and alcohol. The bacteria in the mouth feed off the food we eat, and they are especially attracted to sugar. A plaque forms on the teeth and the bacteria attach to the plaque. Brushing the teeth and rinsing the mouth after eating are important ways of dealing with bad breath. Flossing is also very important. Local treatment, such as breath mints and mouthwashes are only short-term solutions. I find cloves after a meal very useful as a natural breath mint. I also use them for their antibacterial action in order to keep my mouth healthy and also to prevent me from catching bacteria from my patients. The real underlying treatment, however, should be to look at a person's diet to see what they are eating on a regular basis which is causing this bad breath. The most likely thing is sugar, which feeds the bacteria and allows them, in the dark, moist recesses of the mouth, to create types of bacterial odors that can cause bad breath.

Let us consider the function of the tongue. In animals, especially dogs, we know it is an organ of elimination of moisture, much as our skin eliminates perspiration. Perspiration or sweat is not just pure water; it contains salt and by-products of chemical processes in the body, in which waste is excreted by the kidneys, through the intestines and through the skin. The tongue serves the same function, so the body in trying to eliminate waste uses the tongue. It is conceivable that these wastes find their way to the tongue and sometimes coat the tongue, contributing to bad breath. The more waste products and the more toxic the waste products from the body, the more the tongue is coated, and the breath has a foul odor. People who have a very clean diet—by which I mean plenty of fresh vegetables, fruits, nuts, seeds, grains, fish and chicken—rarely have bad breath. People who eat sugar, dairy products, coffee, alcohol and meat tend to have more bad breath. Meat, itself, takes up to seven hours to digest in the intestines.

Most people do not chew their food properly. If you chew properly, then you can digest up to one-third of your carbohydrates right in your mouth. However, meat is a protein, and it requires hydrochloric acid in the stomach for digestion. The reason meat takes seven hours is that it takes that long for enough hydrochloric acid to be built up and to break down the protein molecules. During the seven-hour period, more and more food is taken in and combined with the digesting protein. This leads to gas and fermentation in the stomach which, besides causing belching and flatulence, can bring the odors into the mouth and create bad breath. Similarly, when sugar is put into the stomach and there are other foods in the stomach, there can be a process of fermentation that has the effect of creating alcohol in the stomach and the intestines. This can be easily measured in the bloodstream after the intake of sugar or even of fruit. Please read the chapters on **Digestion, Candidiasis,** and **Food Combining** for more information on this topic.

Bed-Wetting

∂. At a certain age, children are expected to sleep through the night without wetting the bed. This can be anywhere from age two to seven. The causes for bed-wetting are sometimes psychological stress, especially if there is another child born around the time when the older child has been dry at night for several months. The bed-wetting can be an attention-getting device on an unconscious psychological level. Other stresses in the home can result in bed-wetting. Sleep-overs often produce bed-wetters because of the excitement and stress of sleeping over. However, in my practice, I make a point of looking for food allergies that can contribute to irritation or relaxation of the bladder neck muscles which allow the urine to leak during the night. The urination can come during the very deep sleep phase when there is not enough arousal to wake a child up and allow him or her to go to the bathroom. The foods that seem to cause the most problems are milk, orange juice, peanut butter, and sugar, but almost any food can conceivably be a problem. Drinking before bed itself can fill the bladder and create a problem. Limiting food and liquid intake after supper would be appropriate. Also, getting the child up to urinate when the adults are going to bed would help to keep the bladder empty. Please see the chapter on **Allergies** for more information on this topic.

Birth Control

Birth Control Pill

Unfortunately, everyone has become so used to the concept of the birth control pill that this option is often the only one that people equate with birth control. Even though several studies have confirmed that the birth control pill can cause cancer, doctors and drug companies alike refuse to "alarm" the public with these unsavory statistics. The pill, a combination of synthetic female hormones, taken daily, gives the body the impression that it is in a constant state of pregnancy. After the pill is stopped, the return of the normal period is often delayed. The high rate of infertility today may also be related to the pill. Women on the pill suffer a higher rate of strokes and liver disease. It is said that the newer low dose pill has fewer side effects but it has not been tested on an entire generation of individuals as yet. In fact, the whole notion of playing around with our hormones is a gigantic experiment.

If the pill is taken, it should not be taken for more than five years, not beyond the age of 35, and not by women who smoke or who have a family history of female cancer.

Women who take the pill also suffer an increased incidence of Candidiasis (see the chapter on **Candidiasis**), although the symptoms may not appear for several years. Symptoms will be aggravated by intake of antibiotics along with the BCP (antibiotics can also inactivate the BCP). Stress and the intake of a highly refined food diet can also stimulate Candida growth. If a decision is made to take the BCP, the following advice should be followed to prevent side effects. The BCP causes yeast overgrowth due to the increased level of hormones so one should take acidophilus on a regular basis to increase the level of good bacteria in the system. Maintain a healthy diet of whole grains, nuts and seeds, vegetables, fish and chicken and avoid bread with yeast, highly refined foods such as sugar, and cut back on cheese.

Supplements that are necessary when taking the pill include a *B complex* with *B6* and *folic acid*. In some studies, women on the pill experience a type of depression which is due to a deficiency of *vitamin B6*. If there is this side affect, the amount of *B6* should be a minimum of 50 mg per day. *Vitamin C* with *bioflavins* is important for symptoms of gum swelling or bleeding and varicose vein formation, especially the small spidery web-like veins. The dosage would be 1000 mg of *vitamin C* a day with 250 mg of *bioflavins*. *Vitamin E* is also important to help the metabolism of the birth control pill, 200 I.U. per day. *Zinc*, 25 mg per day, is important since it has been found that women on birth control pills have lower levels of zinc. If a woman has side effects on the pill which do not go away even when the pill is discontinued, then homeopathic remedies are useful. The remedy would have to be chosen according to the symptoms and to the constitution of the patient. These might include *Sepia, Pulsatilla* and *Nat. mur.*

Diaphragm

The diaphragm is a barrier method of birth control. This disc-like piece of rubber is fitted by a doctor and inserted by the individual before intercourse. It is heavily coated with a spermicidal gel which acts as the real barrier to the tiny sperm that can wiggle around the edges of the diaphragm. Pregnancy can occur if the gel is not used or if the diaphragm bends and allows the sperm to pass by. Constipation can cause the diaphragm to bend and the pressure on the urethra can cause bladder infections.

Cervical Cap

The cervical cap seems to be a more comfortable and better fitting barrier method. The cap fits on the cervix and is also used with spermicidal jelly. The user must be able to feel the cervix and feel that the cap is attached snugly around the cervix. It has the same problem as the diaphragm in that it can become dislodged and allow the sperm to travel through the cervical canal. The earliest a woman may be aware that there was a failure in contraception is when she misses her next period. The

main side effect from this form of contraception is an un-
wanted pregnancy.

Condoms

Aside from abstinence, the condom is the only birth control
method that will protect you from AIDS and other sexually
transmitted diseases.

Condoms and foam are a double barrier method in which
both partners take responsibility for birth control. The best kind
of condom is one with a reservoir tip which holds the released
sperm so that it does not travel up the sides of the condom and
come in contact with the vagina. One good thing about condoms and foam is that if a sperm or two find their way into
the vagina the foam should kill them. Another good thing about
this method is that if the condom breaks it is immediately apparent. If the woman is mid-cycle, (the time of ovulation and highest fertility) it is possible to take a "morning after pill." This
would consist of six to eight Ovral birth control pills, two taken
as soon as possible and two taken every twelve hours. These
pills cause the lining of the uterus to grow and since the pills
are not continued, the lining is then shed and this makes it
impossible for any implantation to occur.

The side effects of condoms and foam are the potentially irritating effects of the acidifying foam. If used properly and consis-
tently, this is a highly safe method of birth control. The morning
after pill, in bringing on an early period, can obviously throw
off your cycle. Normal cycling should resume in a month or
two. You must be very careful at this time and, if doing natural
birth control, be very aware of your mucus, etc. A homeopathic
remedy can be made from an Ovral pill and used to balance
the side effects of taking it. (See the chapter **Make Your Own
Remedy.**)

Natural Birth Control

By far the safest, most natural and most responsible method of birth control is natural birth control. With this method you study the natural menstrual cycle and measure temperatures and cervical mucus to determine which days you can become pregnant and which days are safe. It can also be used for infertile women to learn the best time to have intercourse. The best resource for this information is Fertility Management, 598 St. Clair Ave. W., Toronto, Ontario, M6C1A6. They have information on resources in the U.S. as well as in Canada.

Bites

⁓ Mosquitoes seem to dislike the odor produced from the ingestion of *B vitamins*, especially *thiamine (B1)*, so in mosquito season, on the advice of your doctor, take extra dosages of the B-Complex, including B1. Most commercial mosquito sprays are strong chemical compounds that might affect one adversely when absorbed, but there is one natural one: a citrus lotion called citronella. This insect repellent should not have any side effects when, or if, absorbed. The latest advice on treating bites is to put a moistened aspirin on the cleaned bite area to relieve the pain and stop the inflammation. Homeopathic remedies for bites and stings include *Apis* and *Ledum*. If someone has a bee-sting allergy, apis can be used every few minutes. However an Anakit (bee-sting kit) should also be handy. This contains adrenalin and a needle, and should be used, especially if the sting is around the face or throat. *Ledum* is a good remedy for spider bites, or even cat and dog bites. These bites can produce an infection, and the area should be cleaned well and should be examined by a doctor, who may advise an antibiotic cream, a tetanus booster, and possibly antibiotics by mouth. Sometimes soaking the wound in an herbal antibiotic, such as *echinacea*, and poulticing with a clay pack, or *comfrey*, or even a bread poultice, can prevent infection from occurring. An infection will produce a red line from the wound toward the nearest lymph node as the body tries to clear the infection, but it often indicates to doctors that an antibiotic should be used. If you use an antibiotic, be sure to take acidophilus bacteria along with it to prevent an overgrowth of Candidiasis.

Bladder Infections

For anyone suffering from chronic or frequent bladder infection, the book *You Don't Have to Live With Cystitis* by Dr. Larrian Gillespie is a wonderful source of information. There are chapters on how to deal with acute and chronic infection; information on the allergic causes of bladder symptoms; and advice on all aspects of bladder and kidney disease. The most common cause of bladder infections in women tends to be post-coital infection. During intercourse, the positioning can be such that the urethra is trapped and irritated. This will cause the urethra to swell. If there is bacteria near the urethra, which can migrate from the bowel area, the urethral inflammation and swelling provide an ideal environment for bacteria to grow. Please check Dr. Gillespie's book for specific details. However, in general, to avoid bladder infections after intercourse, be sure not to create this jamming action with the penis which traps the urethra; just pull back an inch or so if this is happening. Wash before and after intercourse with a neutral pH soap and also urinate before and after intercourse to wash bacteria out of the urethra. Taking a homeopathic remedy called *Staphasagria* 6c or 30c, 4 drops one to two times after intercourse, may prevent infection in susceptible people.

Inserting a diaphragm can also result in bacteria overgrowth. Also, the diaphragm as it rests inside the vagina above the pubic bone cuts off the urethra, irritating it and inhibiting bladder emptying. If the bacteria are not flushed out after intercourse they can overgrow. Tampons may also cause some of the same problems as diaphragms and lead to bladder infections.

If bladder symptoms such as frequent urination, burning and pressure begin, it is important to submit a urine sample to your doctor so that she or he may have it tested for bacterial over-growth. While waiting for results, the natural treatments could include ½ to ¼ tsp of baking soda in one glass of water every 30 minutes. This can help make the urine less acidic and there-fore less burning. Avoid caffeinated tea and coffee and take *pars-ley* or *chamomile* tea in large quantities to help treat the condition. Lots of water is the key to flushing out bacteria. Also homeopathic remedies such as *Cantharis* or *Causticum* in the 6c or 30c potency taken every hour can be helpful. If it is a post-coital irritation, *Staphasagria* 6 or 30 c can be taken every hour.

In young girls, bladder infections can be the result of taking bubble baths, so they should be avoided. Do not take chamo-mile tea with homeopathic remedies; it can neutralize them.

Simple commonsense advice to prevent bladder infections in-cludes avoiding tight jeans, wearing loose cotton underwear, and avoiding scented tampons, pads or even colored toilet paper. After a bowel movement, wipe from front to back to avoid pulling bowel bacteria into the vagina/urethra area.

Studies show that pure cranberry juice or even cranberry tab-lets help bladder infections. If you must take an antibiotic, ask your doctor for a urinary antiseptic such as *nitrofurantoin* or *nalidixic acid* which do not affect the intestinal bacteria and cause Candidiasis. If you have to use an antibiotic, be sure and take yogurt or acidophilus tablets as well. Read the chapters on **Candidiasis** and **Antibiotics**.

Boils

◠ Boils are usually a staphylococcal infection. They can pro-duce a lot of pain and are a considerable nuisance. The medical treatment is usually the use of strong antibiotics. However, until antibiotics are necessary, several natural remedies can be used. Boils usually occur in people who have a zinc deficiency and *zinc* is important for wound healing. The amount would be 25 to 50 mg per day during the infection and 25 mg per day when not infected to prevent recurrence. Zinc is found in sunflower seeds, pumpkin seeds and oysters.

Another possible cause of boils is an overload of toxins in the system which stresses the liver, kidney and colon. Thus the toxins are released through the skin. People who have boils should avoid constipation and read the chapter on **Detoxification** in this book. Boils can be treated with poultices to try to bring the boil to a head and then discharge the contents. Clay, which is available in health food stores, can be prepared and applied to a boil. Poultices of bread moistened with water can be applied to the area or even a hot water compress may bring a boil to a head. If fresh or dry *comfrey* is available, pulverize or chop one tablespoonful, steep in ½ cup boiling water for fifteen minutes, strain, wrap in gauze and apply to boil, covering with plastic wrap. Leave on a maximum of 12 hours per day.

Homeopathic treatments are with oral doses of:

Hepar sulph. 6c which is used to bring boils to a head. *Calc. sulph.* 6c for recurring crops of boils. *Silicia* 6c for boils that are slow to heal. *Sulphur* 6c for burning and itching boils. All remedies are taken 4 drops three times a day.

Herbal tincture of *echinacea* can be used for a person who is toxic and produces boils, 10 to 15 drops three times a day in water. This could be taken orally or used to soak a boil. Other boil soaks are *hypericum* tincture and *calendula* tincture.

Breastfeeding

ॐ A recent article in a breastfeeding publication *Infact* reviewed almost 100 research articles on the importance of breastfeeding. They concluded that the incidence of all types of infections, especially ear infections, was much lower in breast-fed babies.

The keys to perfect and painless breastfeeding are good milk production and proper positioning of the baby. Good milk production is prepared for during the pregnancy by eating an optimum diet, with plenty of vegetables, moderate amounts of fruit, lots of whole grains, beans, seeds and nuts, fish and chicken, and if dairy is not eaten, proper amounts of calcium and magnesium. During pregnancy and breastfeeding, *calcium* should be at a level of 1500 mg per day, and *magnesium* at half that amount. After delivery, immediate breastfeeding will help stimulate breast-milk production. The herbs that are useful in encouraging breast-milk production are *marshmallow root* and *fennel*. Herbs that diminish breast-milk production are *parsley* and *sage*.

Optimal position advocated by La Leche League is holding the baby in one hand, with the buttocks in the hand and also supported against the hip, and the baby's head in the crook of the elbow. The free hand is used to hold the breast from below. The nipple is held against the baby's lower lip, and this stimulates the baby to open the mouth wide. As the mouth opens, pull the baby's whole body quickly toward your body so that the aerola of the breast fits well into the baby's mouth. The nipple itself should be placed deep in the baby's throat. Proper positioning should result in no breast pain, no nipple pain, and no cracked, raw or irritated nipples. This is a common complaint among breastfeeding mothers, but with proper positioning it should not occur.

If the nipples do become irritated, then *vitamin E oil* will help to heal them. Keeping the clothing dry helps, try not to wear anything that will retain moisture around the nipples. Do not use soap to wash the nipples because of the drying effect. Another important aspect of breastfeeding is to avoid plugged ducts, which can lead to mastitis. Examine the breasts every day to determine if there is an area of hardness or inflammation. Immediately put a hot pack (a wet compress, a heating pad or castor oil pack) on the area. Massage the area from the base of the breast, at the chest wall, out toward the nipple. Make sure the baby is allowed to nurse on that side more frequently. Within twenty-four hours, the plugged duct should be clear; however, if the breast gets more inflamed and you have a temperature and feel like you have the flu, then this could be a sign of mastitis. The usual treatment is antibiotics to prevent further complications, such as breast abscess. The treatment here is rest, lots of fluids, and nursing even more frequently. The baby will not be infected, but with the use of antibiotics, the mother and the baby could become more susceptible to Candidiasis. Take plenty of acidophilus bacteria when you must take antibiotics, and watch the baby for oral thrush or diaper rash. Read the chapter on **Candidiasis** about this condition and how it should be treated.

Bronchitis

෴ Bronchitis often begins with a simple cold that develops into a chronic persistent cough. Therefore, the best treatment for bronchitis is to ensure that a cold is not prolonged. See the chapter on **Colds and Flus**. They are most often due to a virus, so antibiotics will not help.

For bronchitis itself, avoidance of mucus-forming foods such as dairy and wheat would be helpful. Lots of fluids are important and mucus-thinning herbs such as *fenugreek*. Use steam or a humidifier to help liquify the mucus. Dehydration is quite common with bronchitis. If your urine output does not equal your water input then you may be becoming dehydrated which can elevate your fever and solidify your mucus.

Bronchial herb tea available in health food stores simply labelled *Bronchial Tea* would include herbs such as *mullein* and *lobelia*, which are useful for this condition. There are many homeopathic remedies for bronchitis. *Bryonia* 6c, 4 drops every few hours, is one of the best. However a full list of remedies would allow you to identify the best remedy for a particular cough. Study the remedies section in this book.

Smoking (or smokers) should be avoided especially since it is the most common reason people get bronchitis. If the cough persists, especially in certain environments, allergies should be a consideration. For those who have a prolonged cough, an allergy to animal dander, dust or mold can be the underlying cause. However, if the condition persists, it would be advisable to have a chest x-ray to make certain there is no underlying pathology. The next modality might be to have acupuncture with a Chinese medical doctor. These doctors can do meridian diagnosis and determine where the energy imbalance is occurring in the body causing this condition. Check locally for doctors in your area that use Chinese medicine.

Bruising

⤵ Bruising usually occurs after an injury, after bumping into a piece of furniture that shouldn't have been there in the first place, or even after running or exercising, which by gravity and impact, can break small capillaries. For bruises caused by an injury, the most important treatment is *Arnica* 30C or 200C by mouth, and *arnica cream* on the bruise, as long as the bruise does not break the skin. Arnica is a mountain plant that was probably first discovered by mountain goats. Arnica is quite amazing for anything from a black eye to a stubbed toe. The more serious the injury, the more frequently the Arnica is taken, anywhere from every 15 minutes to every two hours. Ice is also useful for the first twenty-four or thirty-six hours to stop the inflammation and to stop the inflammatory products from leaching out into the surrounding area and triggering off more inflammation. The ice packs should be applied every 15 to 20 minutes. After thirty-six hours, heat can be used to clear the dead blood cells from the area by increasing the circulation.

Frequent bruising may be due to medication such as aspirin,

or other drugs such as anti-depressants and asthma drugs, which can inhibit platelet aggregation, thereby inhibiting clotting, and leading to even larger bruises. Alcoholics tend to bruise easily because of liver side effects. Other people who bruise easily can have a vitamin C deficiency; it may not be just vitamin C but the bioflavins—a part of the vitamin C complex that are important. Bioflavinoids are useful for varicose veins, hemorrhoids, stroke prevention, heavy menstrual bleeding, as well as for bruising. *Vitamin C*, 500 mg, two or three times a day, along with 250 mg of *bioflavinoids* several times a day will help strengthen the blood vessels. *B12* and *folic acid* are two vitamins responsible for the size of the red blood cell. If these vitamins are deficient then the cell size expands and the membrane weakens and there is bleeding and bruising. A doctor should do blood tests to determine if there is a rare B12 deficiency condition called pernicious anemia. If there is not, and B12 or folic acid are indicated, supplements should be taken.

Burning Feet

ॐ This unusual condition is often very difficult to diagnose. The doctor must rule out impaired circulation, hardening of the arteries, *B12* deficiency or diabetes. Medically, these conditions could be ruled out only when they are in the full-blown state. However, the syndrome may be caused by a mild form of any one of these conditions. Therefore, read the chapter on **Atherosclerosis** and **Diabetes** and be sure to increase the amounts of *B12* in the diet or take supplements. Some doctors may be willing to try *B12* injections for the treatment of this condition. *Vitamin E*, 400 I.U. per day and *calcium* and *magnesium*, about 800 mg per day of each may be needed. The *B-complex*, 50 mg per day for proper nerve nutrition might be useful. Adequate exercise is very important and certainly detoxification can help. (See the chapter on **Detoxification**.) Some people improve by taking epsom salts baths or foot baths. In some cases, diluted cidar vinegar as a foot bath is helpful. Chinese water therapy uses cold water foot baths just prior to retiring for the evening; these are reported to be very good for this particular condition. Each individual will have to explore a variety of these natural methods to determine the best one for him or her.

Burning Mouth

ဢ This condition can be due to food allergies, Candidiasis or vitamin or mineral deficiencies. One should avoid the most common allergens to see if the condition improves. Read the chapters on **Allergies** and **Candidiasis** to determine common allergens. The vitamin and mineral deficiencies could be magnesium, B12, folic acid, iron or zinc. The treatment levels would be 400 mg of *magnesium; B12* by injection, 1,000 mcg per week; *folic acid,* 5 mg daily, now available only with a prescription; *iron,* chelated form 25 mg per day: and *zinc* 25 mg per day. The mineral deficiencies can be assessed through a hair analysis by your doctor or naturopath.

Burns

ဢ The immediate treatment for burns is cold water on the burn and oral ingestion of homeopathic *Cantharis* 6c, 30c or 200c every few minutes. This should be in everyone's first aid kit. You must never break a burn blister because this can allow infection. The burn blister protects the underlying skin while it heals. *Aloe vera gel* or the open leaf from the aloe vera plant can be placed on burns. *Vitamin E* oil is also good for the local treatment of burns and scars after the blister has healed. *Calendula* lotion or *Hypericum* lotion can also be applied. *Homeopathy for the First Aider* by Dr. Dorothy Shepherd belongs in every self-care library. Homeopathic first aid kits are available using the remedies outlined in this book in the **Rem-**

edies section and in the chapter on **First Aid**. See the back page for instructions on ordering.

Bursitis

~ This is a painful condition of the bursa usually of the shoulder but there can be bursitis of any bursa or fluid-filled shock absorber in any joint. With the shoulder, it is often caused by overuse, injury or lying on the shoulder in a painful position for a long period of time such as overnight. The condition is best treated with natural anti-inflammatories (before going to medication). These would be vitamin C and pancreatic enzymes; 1 gram of *vitamin C* three times a day and 2 *pancreatic enzyme* tablets three times a day. Also useful are castor oil packs to decrease the inflammation. Several tablespoons are put on an old cloth or towel and wrapped over the area. Use ice first, especially if the area is inflamed and hot. After two days you may begin to alternate the castor oil packs with ice. Try ten minutes of one and ten minutes of the other.

Rest is important at first. Then begin gentle exercise. The best known exercise is performed by leaning your chest over the end of an ironing board with the painful arm hanging and swing gently back and forth for a few minutes several times a day. Physiotherapy can be helpful using ultrasound or interferential or diathermy treatment.

Acupuncture or laser-acupuncture by a naturopath can also alleviate the condition and a good chiropractor can also be helpful. The longer bursitis is ignored, the more chance it has of becoming chronic.

Callouses and Corns

~ A callous is a build-up of tough skin in an area is that is being subjected to extra pressure and extra work. Callouses on the hands may be from using a hammer all day; callouses on the feet maybe from ill-fitting shoes. If the pressure gets very severe, then a corn can develop. A corn is merely a callous with a hard core. To prevent these callouses and corns, wear proper footgear that does not put pressure on the heels or the toes. Sometimes people will have to wear insoles or special orthotics, which are insoles specially made by podiatrists or chiropractors to keep the foot in the proper position within the shoe.

The recommendation for treating callouses is to soak the feet in various solutions. Epsom salts in warm water is good for relieving the inflammation that can occur due to the callous or corn. Sometimes the corn is located near a bursa, which is a small sack of lubricating fluid that is found between every joint in the body. The epsom salts will help take down this inflammation. To remove the callous, the best remedy I've found is to cut a leaf from an aloe vera plant that is the same size as the corn or callous, slice the leaf down the center so that the interior gel can be placed against the callous, and then cover with several Band-Aids. This can be worn to bed, and in the morning the callous or corn can be rubbed off with a dry face cloth or perhaps a pumice stone. If the callouses are around the heel, then you have thick, cracked skin. An excellent soak is half-and-half vinegar and castor oil. This can be kept in an old pot and reheated as needed. It's a very messy solution, but it works wonders—after soaking, preferably near a tub, wash off the material and use a pumice stone to smooth away the dead skin. Podiatrists advise people with pressure areas between the toes to put toe pads made of foam between the toes, or to use lambs' wool between the toes. The best way, as mentioned before, to avoid corns and callouses is to choose proper footwear.

Cancer

ᔕ This is a topic that I study more and more. We are all aware of the causes of cancer: smoking and second-hand smoke in lung cancer; high fat, low fiber, high red meat diet in colon cancer and breast cancer; radiation and chemical exposure in leukemia; and general poor diet and excessive stress in all forms of cancer. In fact, reliable sources now are documenting that up to 85% of all cancer is environmentally induced.

The paralysis that overcomes a person when he or a family member is diagnosed with cancer often causes an automatic adherence to the conventional methods of cancer treatment with surgery, chemotherapy and radiation.

I have always thought that prevention of cancer is the best policy. People with a strong family history of cancer should read about cancer therapy and alternatives now and choose methods that will prevent cancer or have in mind the modalities they will use in conjunction with conventional therapy if they are diagnosed with cancer in the future. Two excellent books which describe alternative and complementary cancer treatments are *Cancer Therapy: An Independent Consumer's Guide to Non-Toxic Treatment and Prevention* by Ralph W. Moss, Ph.D. and *Options: The Alternative Cancer Treatment Book* by Richard Walters.

The psychoneuroimmunology connection to illness is extremely important. People should recognize that negative thoughts bring negative consequences and positive thoughts bring positive consequences. Mind enhancing techniques like the Silva Method can be invaluable for people to mobilize all their healing energies all the time for optimum health and to prevent illness.

Candidiasis

This condition has been newly titled Candidiasis Related Syndrome because it is a complex of different etiologies, symptoms and treatments. Year by year we are finding more people affected by Candida overgrowth. The yeast, Candida Albicans always has lived in the gastrointestinal tract but under the influence of antibiotics, the birth control pill, cortisone, a highly refined bread and sugar diet, and stress, the yeast are encouraged to overgrow and their toxins and their byproducts can adversely effect the whole body.

The symptoms range from headaches, head congestion, depression and anxiety to throat and chronic cold symptoms, swollen glands, coated tongue, gastric upset, gas and bloating, constipation or diarrhea, vaginitis, arthritis, cystitis, muscle and joint aches and numbness and tingling of the extremities. The symptoms are so widespread, it is sometimes difficult for an individual or her doctor to even comprehend that it could be a symptom complex.

It is important to read the books on Candidiasis: *The Yeast Syndrome* by John Trowbridge, M.D., *The Yeast Connection* by William Crook, M.D., or *The Missing Diagnosis* by Orian Truss M.D. It is only through reading and understanding the syndrome that people can relate it to their individual problems.

The best diagnosis for this condition is now available by special culture and anti-fungal drug sensitivity testing and blood antibody tests to the Candida. With these scientific tests, doctors are able to diagnose and treat each person individually.

The anti-Candida program is not a simple one and often well-trained counsellors are required to help implement it. The treatment usually begins with a diet which is very strict for the first few weeks: avoiding sugar, bread with yeast, fruit, fermented foods and often most grains. The person has some idea by the end of this period whether the dietary restriction is working. Most people with Candidiasis report that they begin to feel much better by the second or third week. The first week can present some aggravation of symptoms if the yeast that are dying off flood the system. After several weeks on a strict diet, a gradual reintroduction of foods would indicate whether problems with specific foods still exist, either because of food allergy or yeast sensitivity.

Sometimes it is necessary to have food allergy testing to determine specific allergies. The next step while waiting for the test results is to add *acidophilus* bacteria to your diet. Acidophilus is a good bacteria that helps build up the normal flora in the bowel as the yeast are being killed off. Supplements are available in health food stores.

The next steps include eating anti-fungal foods such as *garlic* or taking two to three garlic capsules daily. *Pau d'Arco* (also called *La Pacho* or *Taheebo*) tea is also helpful.

If the Candida testing shows a moderate to high level of yeast growth, then antifungal medications are begun; either *caprylic acid* made from coconut oil or *nystatin* or *Nizoral*. Caprylic acid comes in tablet and capsule form. The capsules seem to help kill yeast in the upper gastrointestinal tract and the tablets affect the yeast in the lower GI tract. Most people have to take a combination of the two. These are begun very gradually to ensure there are no side effects and working up to a combination of three capsules and three tablets a day before meals. The nystatin is a prescription medication with seemingly few side effects. The dosage is 500,000 units four times a day before meals. Powder form is best (the pink tablets by Lederle or the coated tablet by Squibb known as Mycostatin make good substitutes). The coating on the Mycostatin may help keep the medication stabilized until it travels to the lower part of the GI tract. Some people simply wash off the chocolate colored coating and use this tablet. I consider nystatin powder the best because it can be used by mouth as a gargle for the local thrush in the mouth and when swallowed it can treat the yeast in the upper gastrointestinal tract. It can be used as a vaginal douche and in a rectal suspension to get at the yeast in the vagina and more importantly in their reservoir, the gut. Also people can dilute the powder and use as nose drops or even ear drops. Nizoral is taken 200 mg one-half to one tablet twice a day. It does have reported side effects of liver toxicity, especially in very sensitive or very ill people so it is necessary to perform liver function tests every four to six weeks if the patient is on long-term treatment.

A recent book on the immune system suggests that nystatin is not a good drug for Candida without explaining why. The author, when asked, said that it was because nystatin does not go into the blood. However, this is precisely why I use nystatin first because it does not go into the blood and put a strain on the liver. And most importantly, we are not dealing with systemic Candidiasis in the blood, we are dealing with mucocutaneous Candidiasis located in the mucus membranes and skin. The idea behind treatment is to control the reservoir of yeast which lives in the bowel so that it will not overgrow, and to use methods to enhance the growth of good bacteria and enhance the immune system to take care of itself. The medical model of using the strongest drug on the block to knock out the bad guys does not work.

In my experience, using only one or two of the above methods, no matter how much you use or how strict you are, will not irradicate the yeast. Nor in my opinion, will homeopathic remedies work alone on Candida. In fact, remedies for constitutional treatment have even less chance of working if there is unsuspected yeast overgrowth which is not treated properly. By properly, I mean all the above steps done in moderation. I am not saying cure because there will always be some yeast in our bodies with the possibility of overgrowth with the right conditions. And again, if the standard dosage of an antifungal does not work, it is not necessary to increase the dosage more and more but to use the medication in other ways, do all the above steps and investigate other possibilities.

There are many intricacies in the treatment of Candidiasis. One has to treat yeast as well as look for and treat hypoglycemia, Epstein-Barr, food allergies, hypothyroidism, stress and PMS. Therefore, the best advice is to seek counselling with persons who are knowledgeable about these conditions who can spend the time sorting out the problems. Unfortunately, doctors can ill afford the luxury of spending the required hour or more helping patients with these complex situations. Therefore, the patient must take responsibility for researching and educating herself as to what to do, in conjunction with direction from the doctors and Candida counsellor, to try and achieve optimum health. There are many pieces of advice and information that have been used for individual cases that are too numerous to note but I would refer you to the Candida Research and Information Foundation newsletter which contains the latest news and information available on various immune system topics. There are branches in Canada and the U.S.

Canker Sores

☙ The most common causes of canker sores in the mouth are: an overload of acidic foods in the diet, hot foods, damage to the inside of the mouth due to biting or toothbrush injury. Acidic foods would include fruits, tomatoes, chewable vitamin C and chocolate. A mechanical imbalance of the biting surface of the teeth can lead to accidental biting at the sides of the inner cheek and cause trauma that will lead to cankers. Also food allergies and Candidiasis can cause cankers. Read the chapters on **Allergies** and **Candidiasis**.

The treatment of cankers is to avoid acidic foods and use *acidophilus* or *yogurt* to restore normal bacterial flora in the mouth. Rinsing the mouth with *dilute hydrogen peroxide, goldenseal tea,* or *myrrh tea* can relieve the symptoms. Dabbing the canker with *alum* can relieve some of the pain. Cankers can be difficult to heal because the mouth is always moist and you cannot get a healing salve to stick to the canker.

Cankers are another condition where people have to play detective to determine what they were doing just prior to developing that last canker sore and to determine whether there is a direct correlation. Homeopathic *Boric acid* 6c can be used for this condition. Some people have reported that their canker sores diminished after appropriate treatment for candidiasis.

Carpal Tunnel Syndrome

☙ The carpal tunnel is the area of the wrist where tendons, nerves and blood vessels go from the forearm to the hand. It is on the palm side of the wrist, and there is a band of tissue across this tunnel that can become swollen. The tendons in the wrist, especially if this band is swollen, can become inflamed. People who are subject to this condition tend to use their wrists a lot and with repetitive motions, such as in hammering, knitting, typing, writing, and massaging. The tendon can swell up, putting pressure on the nerve that runs into the hand and the result can be numbness and tingling of the fingers, the feeling that the hand is falling asleep, and a lot of pain. Pregnant women are very susceptible to this condition. Twice as many women as men suffer from carpal tunnel syndrome. While one hand is usually symptomatic, both hands can suffer.

Medically, there is a surgical procedure to release the band over the tendons, but it doesn't cure the problem. Exercises include elevating the hands to decrease pressure on the nerve, gently rotating the wrists in circular motions, and massaging the fingers, palms, and up the wrists toward the elbows with the hand held upright. Sometimes it's merely a matter of cutting back on the amount of work you do with your hands.

Ice and cold packs will decrease the inflammation in the wrist, and proper sleep posture is very important. Don't lie on your arm at night and don't allow your hands to be in a lower position than the rest of your body. Physiotherapists can fit wrist splints to alleviate the condition. However, the best treatment that I have found over the years is high-dose *vitamin B6* therapy. Dr. John Ellis has been treating carpal tunnel syndrome for years, and he believes that this syndrome is actually caused by a deficiency of vitamin B6. The dosage is anywhere from 50 mg to 350 mg per day. The symptoms can take from four to eight weeks to begin to subside, but in my experience, there is relief with this treatment. There have been reports of people self-medicating with B6 at 2,000 mg and causing numbness and tingling of the nerves; however, up to 400 mg is thought to be safe, and even for people using 2,000 mg, the symptoms subsided upon stopping the medication. I would recommend a B-Complex along with the B6 to prevent an imbalance from using one B vitamin alone.

Other recommendations would be *calcium* and *magnesium* for the pain and the nervous system, and possibly *vitamin B12* injections to provide treatment for the nerves. A *multiple vitamin and mineral* supplement might also be useful. For overweight women who have this condition, I would recommend a weight-reduction program.

Another possible cause might be food allergies leading to fluid retention, which then swells up the band of skin covering the carpal tunnel. Please read the chapter on **Allergies**.

Cataracts

٤. This condition is caused by a thickening and cloudiness of the lens of the eye. Some people feel this is due to a toxicity in the body and a build up of oxidation products in the lens of the eye. Microwave radiation has been known to cause cataracts, so be careful of microwave ovens. The substances that will detoxify and prevent these oxidation products are *bioflavins*, 500–1,000 mg per day; *vitamin E*, 400–800 mg per day; *calcium and magnesium* in a 1:1 ratio, 500 mg of each per day; *B complex*, 50 mg once or twice a day; *vitamin C*, 1,000 mg one to three times a day.

Chronic Fatigue Syndrome

٤. (See Epstein-Barr)

Cold Extremeties

٤. This is often due to poor circulation, yet there are many people who experience this condition who exercise heavily. Other reasons might be low thyroid or low blood sugar. Please refer to the chapters on these two conditions under **Hypothy-roidism** and **Hypoglycemia**.

Cold Sores

ɔ This condition is also called Herpes I. The herpes virus, both orally or in the genital region, sits on the nerve root underneath the skin and will be reactivated under times of stress: in women, premenstrually when the hormones are elevated or if stimulated by sun or heat. The treatment is to avoid stress, too much sun on the skin, and to maintain an excellent diet, good exercise and sleep habits.

Prevention includes using a sun block such as zinc ointment on the lips. Zinc solution at the beginning of the tingling stage can speed healing. So can ice applied to the area or witch hazel or alcohol to decrease inflammation and help dry it up. You may have to boil or replace your tooth brush after the blister stage so you won't be reinfected. Most people find that two days after their cold sore is at a peak, another one pops up nearby.

When cold sores appear, the treatment can begin with lysine, an amino acid which retards the production of RNA, which is the building block of viruses. *Lysine* is taken in 500 mg capsules two capsules three times a day. The foods that contain lysine are fish, chicken, lamb, milk, cheese, beans, brewers yeast, bean sprouts, fruit and vegetables. Eat as much of these foods as possible during an outbreak. Arginine is an amino acid which can lower the levels of lysine. Therefore, cut down on these foods: carob, chocolate, gelatin, coconut, oats, soy beans, peanuts, wheat germ, and whole wheat flour. It is not that they are bad foods but just the wrong balance of amino acids during this condition. In fact, if your diet is mostly arginine-containing foods and you are subject to herpes outbreaks, then it would be a good idea to stop them for a while and see if your condition improves.

The best supplements to boost the immune system to treat

herpes are *B6, B12, folic acid, pantothenic acid,* all available together in a *B complex,* 50 mg 1 to 2 per day. *Calcium and magnesium, selenium,* and *zinc* may be taken in a mineral complex; *vitamin A* and *vitamin E* can be found in a *multiple vitamin complex.*

The homeopathic remedy for cold sores and also for genital sores is *Herpes* 200c, 4 drops three times a day for three days only during an outbreak. The next remedy is *Natrum mur.* 6c, 4 drops three times a day to be taken for one week after finishing the three days of *Herpes* 200c. Many people have found relief and if not a cure, certainly a decrease in outbreaks by using this treatment.

If there is a stress pattern or particular timing to your herpes, take lysine and more supplements around those times.

Colds and Flus

☙ Remember these conditions are the body's way of eliminating mucus. They are usually preceded by excessive eating or poor eating habits, lack of rest, overwork, worry or temperature changes as in fall and spring. First of all, eat wholesome foods and get enough rest. At the onset of seasonal weather changes, take hot and cold showers to acclimatize the skin. Short 30 second blasts of cold will do.

If a cold or flu begins: don't fight it, don't get mad, and go to bed for a day or two.

- Stop all sugar, dairy and wheat intake to decrease mucus and don't eat heavy foods like meat.
- Don't smoke.
- Take plenty of fruit and vegetable juices and chicken broth.
- If there are not contraindications, use an enema with the juice of one lemon to pull out toxins.
- Take epsom salts baths, two cups in hot water to open pores.

- Wrap up warm to encourage sweating and wrap a scarf around your throat.
- Wear a hat at all times to avoid the possible loss of 40% of body heat.
- Use a vaporizer; mucus can collect at night if the air is too dry.
- Do chest clapping to loosen mucus in the chest.
- Take supplements such as *vitamin C*, 4 to 10 grams and *vitamin A*, 30,000 I.U. daily and suck on zinc lozenges.

Herbs useful for a cold are: *sage tea* for cough (steep 20 minutes); *fenugreek tea* for mucus (steep 5 minutes); *ginger* grated and boiled, 2 tablespoons in three cups of water, gargle and use as poultice by saturating a hand towel and wrapping around the throat, changing when poultice becomes cool. Use *goldenseal, garlic* or *echinacea* herbal antibiotics as tincture, tablets or teas at least three times a day; *mullein* and *lobelia* for chest congestion, ½ teaspoon each in teas three times a day. These herbs can also be used as a chest poultice for pleurisy, pneumonia or bronchitis.

Of course, if a painful sore throat or a cough persists, phone the doctor and get a throat swab or sputum culture to identify bacteria which may require antibiotics. When taking antibiotics, always take *yogurt* tablets or *acidophilus*, both of which are found in health food stores. These replace the good bacteria that the antibiotics kill.

To prevent germs from spreading to others, cover your mouth when coughing, don't use cloth handkerchiefs and wash your hands before touching other people or their possessions. Also, replace or boil your toothbrush so you won't reinfect yourself.

For homeopathic remedies for colds, please study the section in this book on **Remedies** or obtain a book by M. D. Panos called *Homeopathic Remedies at Home*.

The most common cold remedies are *Gelsemium* 6 or 30c, 4 drops every two hours for colds and flus due to overwork and exhaustion, and *Dulcamara* 6c or 30c, every two hours for colds and flus developing at the end of summer and into fall. *Aconite* can be used for the first signs of a cold or flu. *Ferrum phos.* is also used for the beginning of a cold. *Kali bich.* is used for colds and sinusitis with tough stringy mucus. *Hepar sulph.* is used for a left-sided sore throat with a cold. *Pulsatilla* is used for a cold with thick yellow mucus.

The post-influenza sequelae are becoming just as important as the original flu itself. In a recent homeopathic newsletter, Dr. Ben Goldberg lists some remedies that I will pass along.

For Gastrointestinal Symptoms

Antimonium crudum: For digestive upsets from the flu. Thickly coated white tongue, aversion to food, worse from eating, worse with acidic or sour drinks. Fullness in the abdomen.

Kali bich.: Catarrhal complications. Poor digestion, anorexia but craves beer.

Baptisia: After the "stomach flu."

For Asthenia, Lethargy and Weakness

Aurum metallicum: Depression, weakness, hopelessness, brooding, melancholy. Thoughts of suicide, easily annoyed.

Cadmium metallicum purum: A newly proven remedy for severe post-flu depression.

Cocculus indica: Mental and physical despair, slow recovery. Anorexia, insomnia, empty feeling. Sick headaches. Aggravated by motion which may cause nausea and vomiting.

Picric acid: Inability to think, as it causes headaches. Patient lies around as the least mental or physical exertion causes extreme weakness.

Phosphoric acid: Debility and mental exhaustion, poor recovery with weakness, indifference, apathy.

Kali phos.:   Used by some physicians as a general "pick-me-up" for the depleted state following a viral illness.

Carbo. veg.:   Carries the reputation of treating "persons who have never recovered from the effects of some previous illness."

Scutellaria: For nervous weakness after influenza, called nervous fear.

Colic

ᴥ This is a condition of smooth muscle spasm in the intestinal tract of infants. During a colic attack, carry the infant face down along your forearm with its head in your hand and its legs astride your elbow. This puts comforting pressure on its rumbling abdomen.

Colicky babies may need to be burped more than most and doing so relieves gas buildup. In fact, any rhythmic kind of motion either in a car, a swing or being carried seems to give some relief.

Colic is also related to the stress and anxiety of the parents. A baby picks up on their nervousness immediately so parents under stress should seek help.

The formula may be at fault or, if the infant is being breast-fed, colic may be caused by the mother's diet. Breastfeeding mothers should avoid dairy products and any foods that are bitter or gas forming. If this does not relieve symptoms, the baby can be given a dilute tea or tincture of *catnip* or *fennel*; fresh *parsley tea* can also be used, the dosage is 1 teaspoon of the herb to 2 cups of boiling water and let steep for 15 to 20 minutes. Give this to the infant in small teaspoons full when cool.

The homeopathic remedies are *Chamomilla* 6c, 4 drops every

few hours for fussiness and irritability. *Aethusa* 6c is used for colic from sensitivity to breast milk; give this three times a day. *Magnesium carbonate* 6c and *Magnesium phosphate* 6c can be used for colic which seems to be better with heat and pressure, 4 drops three times a day. If symptoms persist, seek the advice of a doctor or pediatrician to make sure there is nothing more serious going on.

Colitis

Colitis is a condition of bowel diarrhea and inflammation. The causes in natural medicine are attributed to improper food digestion. This could mean food sensitivities or allergies or a less-than-perfect diet which can cause bowel irritation. The most common cause is excess wheat or dairy in a person who is unable to digest these foods. Cigarettes, alcohol, coffee, tea, sorbitol and aspartame sweeteners are also implicated.

Dietary treatment is usually begun after a person has had a complete workup to determine whether there are any anatomical problems in the bowel. If the specialist finds nothing anatomically wrong with them, they may be given a diagnosis of mild colitis or irritable bowel. Then it would be wise to seek out nutritional advice. Usually an excellent diet that excludes wheat, dairy, sugar, tea, coffee and red meat is suggested. This diet must be maintained for a minimum period of one month to determine if foods are causing the symptoms.

Most often people are much improved on this regimen. If this is not the case, or if only minor improvement is noted, usually more foods are avoided and, in some cases, food allergy tests are required to determine the culprit foods. These tests are available in a number of labs across the U.S. A new book by Elaine Gottschall called *Food and the Gut Reaction* proposes that the underlying cause of intestinal inflammation and irritation is the improper breakdown of carbohydrates. Her "Specific Carbohydrate Diet" excludes all grains for at least a year and cites anecdotal successes. It is used for ulcerative colitis as well as Crohn's disease. It should be read by anyone with colitis.

A lactose tolerance test can determine a lactose allergy but will not indicate an allergy to any other constituents of milk. The best advice is to eliminate milk for at least two to three weeks to see if there is a change. A person can also be allergic to wheat and this is often due to the gluten in wheat. However, gluten is also found in oats, rye and barley. This means all four grains should be entirely eliminated for at least a month and then challenged back with several meals of gluten grains to determine if reintroduction causes more symptoms. We are also finding a lot of people with symptoms of colitis or irritable bowel who have an overgrowth of Candida in their system. **Candidiasis** must be treated. Please read this chapter.

Some people are affected by too much fiber in the diet. Often a person trying to change their lifestyle and diet and become a healthier person will find that eating "lots" of 100% whole grain breads and grains can cause gas cramps and diarrhea. It may be just a case of too much roughage and gas-forming food that the body isn't used to. Go easy and use psyllium, a gentle stool bulking agent, and lots of water. Fiber actually treats colitis and irritable bowel.

Keep a food diary. Take yogurt or *acidophilus* to build up the good bacteria in the intestines.

Food-combining is often very helpful in calming down irritable bowel. This type of diet has you eating only one to two types of food at a time so your digestion is not stressed. The simple rules are:

1. Eat fruit alone.
2. If you eat protein such as meat, fish, chicken, eggs, cheese, eat it with leafy salad vegetables only.
3. If you eat grains or bread, eat with root vegetables and beans.

Sometimes, in spite of numerous dietary interventions, medications and doctors visits, the symptoms remain. Consider seeing a specialist in behavior modification. You may have developed a behavior pattern of having diarrhea and cramps under stress and you have many triggers that perpetuate the problem. Each time you worry "what if there's no washroom where I'm going, what if I can't get through my presentation," you set off your intestinal muscles, and cramps and diarrhea result. Just as your body learned how to create these symptoms, you can unlearn them. Also check the section on **Candidiasis**.

Constipation

⮞ This condition has been alluded to in several previous chapters and will again be referred to in the chapter on **Detoxification**. Constipation can result for many reasons from poor bowel habits that have been learned at an early age (e.g., young children who fail to evacuate the bowels when they have the urge). Over time, the bowel message to evacuate is lost and the feces have to build up and cause greater and greater stimulation before evacuation occurs. Sometimes it could be as simple as the child not wanting to interrupt play to go to the bathroom. Parents should encourage regular bowel habits. Over time this condition can become more serious and chronic.

One to three bowel movements a day is normal. It is the lack of fiber in our diets that makes us so sluggish. Some consider a bowel movement every three to four days normal, but this is a very dangerous concept to entertain. The longer undigested or discarded food matter remains in the large intestine, the more it putrifies and creates harmful wastes which can be reabsorbed into the blood stream. When you are constipated, you can get a headache. Why would you get pressure from a remote part of your body? There is no direct pressure but the irritation from absorbed poisons. Some of these poisons are carcinogenic.

The cause of constipation can also include sensitivity to certain foods such as dairy. If you drink a lot of milk, avoid it for a few weeks and see what happens.

Medications including antidepressants, codeine, certain calcium supplements and aluminum antacids are constipating. Always take calcium with magnesium, and drink more water. Try to avoid the other medications.

In order to treat this condition, lots of fiber should be ingested. The types of fiber are wheat, oat and rice bran, vegetables, whole grains, nuts and seeds. *Psyllium seed powder* or capsules can be added for extra bulk plus lots of water. The dosage is 1 teaspoon shaken in 8 ounces of water and then an additional 8 ounces of water is taken; this is done twice a day. A little juice can be added for taste. Two extra glasses of water a day can increase the bowel movements. If you use psyllium and do not use extra water, you can actually cause constipation. Castor oil packs can be placed on the abdomen to help stimulate lymphatic circulation of the bowel. Massage can be used; massage of the large intestine is done by massaging upwards on the abdomen on the right side of the body across to just above the umbilicus and downward on the left side of the body.

Exercise is very important for helping speed up bowel transit time. To find out how long it takes to get food from mouth to anus, have a large meal of beets. Your urine might even turn pink and watch for a purple stool. Most calls to doctors' offices about blood in the stool are really due to beets.

There are many homeopathic remedies for constipation. These can be used for a short term to stimulate the body's own vital force to change this condition. A constant ineffectual urging to have a bowel movement is present in people who need the remedy called *Nux vomica*. This remedy is also used when the stool does occur and it is incomplete and unsatisfactory, as though some were left behind. This can be taken 6c, 4 drops two to three times a day for two or three weeks to see if symptoms improve. This remedy is also useful to antidote purgative medicines that have long been used to treat constipation. If the 6c potency seems to be slightly effective, the dosage can be increased or the potency can be increased to 30c or even 200c for a short duration such as a week at most. Use 30c, two to three times a day or 200c, one dose per week.

Sulphur can be used alternating with *Nux vomica*. Sulphur treats ineffectual urging to stool with a sensation of heat and discomfort in the rectum and an uneasy feeling all through the intestinal tract due to gas and bloating. The stools are hard, dry, dark and expelled with great straining and often with great pain. It can also be constipation alternating with diarrhea. The dosage should be of a 30c potency but only used for a few weeks at a time, 4 drops two to three times a day. The most commonly used remedies are *Alumina, Bryonia, Lycopodium, Natrum mur.* and *Graphites.* They should be studied to see if they fit your symptoms.

Dandruff

Dandruff is a very common condition. It is due to buildup of skin cells on the scalp related to excessive oiliness of the scalp. The recommendations are to shampoo the hair every day. If over-the-counter dandruff shampoos are used, rotate them: some loosen the flaky skin, some are antibacterial, some decrease the rate at which the skin cells of the scalp reproduce, and the tar-base actually retards cell growth. I find that when people eat a healthy diet, which includes plenty of vegetables, fruit, whole grains, nuts, seeds, fish and chicken, they rarely have dandruff. The supplements that seem to help the skin, hair and nails include *flax seed oil*, which can be taken in salads or on hot cereals, *evening primrose oil* (3 or 4 capsules per day), *zinc* (25 mg per day), the *B-Complex* (50 mg, 1 or 2 per day), *vitamin A* (10,000 units per day), *cod liver oil* (1 tablespoon per day) and a *multiple vitamin and mineral* supplement.

The natural rinses for the hair include using apple cider vinegar after a shampoo (¼ cup into a pint of warm water). This solution returns the natural acid mantle of the scalp and seems to retard dandruff. *Thyme tea* has an effect on scalp dandruff; it has antibacterial properties. Make a solution of thyme tea in a quart of water using several tablespoons of thyme; boil for one hour, strain, and use one cup of the tea over the hair as a rinse after shampooing. Leave on the hair and don't rinse off.

Remember that dandruff may just be a symptom of a more general imbalance in the body, and in order to treat any symptom, we must consider treating the whole body.

Depression

೨ Depression can have multiple causes and multiple treatments. As in all other conditions, I consider it important for nutrition, proper vitamin supplementation, exercise and sleep to form the basis for any natural approach. Frequently, people with a major stress or grief will find that they are unable to sleep and will stop exercising and stop eating properly. This becomes a vicious cycle of improper care for their body and can prolong the condition or deepen the depression.

Try not to get too discouraged about feeling low because it will only make you feel worse. Try to exercise or go out and do something fun, especially with other people. Sharing your dreams with a friend or counsellor can often help you understand why you're depressed. You may be stuck somehow or you may be in conflict. Talking about it usually helps.

Adolescent depression can accompany the normal youth rebellion. This rebellion often takes the form of not following the parental guidelines for diet, sleep and exercise. Young people eat a large amount of refined foods, fast foods, sugar and general junk food. This can create a relative zinc deficiency in the system and low amounts of zinc can cause mood changes. Also, high sugar intake can deplete vitamin C and the B vitamins which are necessary for proper mood balance. If young people take supplements, get enough sleep, exercise and have a good diet, they can often reverse the symptoms of minor depression.

After pregnancy, women may suffer from postpartum depression. This can be treated with high doses of *zinc*, 50 mg daily for one month, then 25 mg daily. Also *Ignatia* 6c, a homeopathic remedy for postpartum depression is extremely useful. The usual dosage is 4 drops three times a day. The *B vitamins*, 50 mg one or two times a day and *multiple vitamins* as well as *calcium* and *magnesium* in equal ratio about 800 mg of each per day can be helpful. It is important to continue these supplements while breast-feeding for proper nutrition.

Other reasons for depression can include cerebral allergies from food or chemical sources, hypothyroidism, hypoglycemia and Candidiasis. Please read the chapters on these topics to familiarize yourself with these conditions.

Detoxification

The importance of detoxification has been mentioned in several chapters. The body releases waste products through the kidney, bowel and skin. It becomes fairly easy to spot someone who is toxic by poor skin color, puffiness or greasiness of the skin, a lack of luster in the eyes and a general sluggish, apathetic appearance. People may not realize that they are toxic because they have been slowly poisoning themselves and have forgotten what it feels like to be in optimum health.

As you improve your diet and lifestyle, you will go through a detoxification process that can include withdrawal headaches as coffee, alcohol and cigarettes are eliminated. You may also experience an aggravation of symptoms when you go back to old habits. In other words, once the body is able to feel better, if toxic substances are ingested, the body may have a severe reaction to these substances and an immediate feedback should warn you to avoid them. This is in fact a good sign; this is the way the body encourages us to avoid these substances.

A good diet of fresh whole grains, nuts and seeds, vegetables, fruit, fish and chicken will help the body eliminate the toxins from the previous diet. After a regimen of good diet, exercise and sufficient sleep have been implemented and maintained for a minimum of one month, a person can begin short fasts on vegetable broths and vegetable juices as well as using *psyllium seed powder* or *capsules* to increase the bowel movements while on the fast. The *psyllium* is taken 2 capsules twice a day with 2 glasses of water or 1 teaspoon of *psyllium powder* in a jar of water with a bit of fruit juice for taste. This should be shaken vigorously and taken with another glass of water to create the optimum bulking action of the psyllium. The juice fasting can be done for a three-day period every two to three months. This gives the body a good rest from digestion, and toxins which are held in fat storage have a chance to be eliminated. Some people suggest *aloe vera gel* be taken on a regular basis for cleansing. This substance is good for healing the intestines and to detoxify; 1 tablespoon in juice every morning. In special conditions, enemas may be recommended for more thorough cleansing.

Diabetes

ᔧ Diabetes is a condition of high blood sugar. When it occurs in children, it is usually due to damage of the islet cells of the pancreas, perhaps due to a virus. The islet cells produce insulin and without insulin, the blood sugar rises without control. Insulin allows the blood sugar to enter the cells to be used for energy.

Most diabetes, however, is found in adults, often from an overuse of sugar or sometimes by eating allergic foods throughout one's life. The insulin is either overworked or overused and is no longer effective in pushing blood sugar into the cells. The best treatment for diabetes is obviously prevention. When one maintains a well-balanced diet, avoiding sugar and refined foods, the blood sugar is maintained at an even level throughout the day and there is no extra demand for insulin. On the other hand, if one eats a lot of refined foods and sugar throughout the day, the blood sugar becomes elevated and more insulin is required to deal with this extra surge of glucose.

In many instances, diabetes can be acquired due to specific

food allergies. These allergies can create an elevated blood sugar which causes the same strain on the insulin supplies of the body. Therefore, good allergy testing is suggested for those people who have already developed diabetes. The other usual recommendations for diabetic control are weight loss, exercise and avoidance of alcohol and smoking.

Recently, short-sighted researchers have been trying to prove that a diabetic's blood sugar can stay in control even when eating refined sugar in moderate amounts. If these people are being injected with insulin then sugar indeed will be properly metabolized but the point of health and natural medicine is to avoid drugs and medicines. If avoiding sugar accomplishes this (which it does), then that is the most logical first step.

I have personal experience with my father, who developed adult onset diabetes after surgery due to stress. I told him to avoid wheat and, when he did, his blood sugar was normal. After a second surgery the next year, he fell into the hands of a hospital dietician who put him on a diabetic diet which allowed six slices of bread a day! Since he loves bread, he went right ahead. His blood sugar got higher and higher and he ended up on diabetic pills. When I urged him to go off the bread again, his blood sugar returned to normal. If you assume diabetes is incurable and you need pills or drugs for it and you do not want to change your diet, then these scientists are playing your song. However, if you want to get your body back to health, avoid sugar. Take blood glucose tests after you eat a meal containing bread, dairy, vegetables and fruit, You will see what foods your body reacts to and be able to cut down on foods that cause the blood glucose to shoot up.

Another major marker for diabetes and the organ damage it causes is incubation time. It is not just today's blood sugar under ideal lab conditions that is important but the five to twenty year incubation time of using refined sugar. Native populations who have switched to a Western refined and sugar-laden diet developed diabetes after 20 years without exception.

I have personally seen the kidney dialysis machines in Indian villages where the diet is mainly white bread and white sugar, and diabetes has wiped out kidney function. I am not convinced that you can safely eat sugar at all. Sugar is also the main contributor to Candida overgrowth, a condition which plagues diabetics.

The best diet for diabetics includes daily portions of dried peas and beans, whole grains, bran, lots of vegetables, fish, chicken and some fruit. If you are not used to cooking dried beans, be sure to soak them for 12 to 24 hours replacing the water several times to remove the gas-causing substances.

The supplements for diabetes include *chromium*, which has a glucose tolerance factor; the *B complex* and *B12* injections to heal the nerve damage caused by the excess sugar; *vitamin C* to fight infection, and wound healing; *zinc* for wound healing in the gluconate or picolinate form; *calcium* and *magnesium* in a 1-to-1 ratio; and for the Candida overgrowth caused by the excess sugar, use *garlic* as an antifungal and *acidophilus* which is the good bowel bacteria.

Diaper Rash

(SEE BABY TIPS)

Diarrhea

⮑ For more information on this topic, read the chapter on **Colitis.** Diarrhea in general can occur due to infection from bacterial sources, viral sources or parasites, and is often called gastroenteritis. Or it can be due to food poisoning or food allergies. With an acute onset of diarrhea, it is important to have stool tests performed in a laboratory for proper diagnosis. Also see a doctor immediately if there is blood in the stool. There are several medical treatments for diarrhea. If there is no organism identified, or while waiting for diagnosis, the individual can begin by trying the following program:

೨1) Avoid all dairy products because the enzymes for the digestion of dairy are usually flushed out or otherwise unavailable. Thus, these foods can be irritating to the bowel and may prolong the diarrhea.

೨2) Avoid citrus and acidic fruits which can irritate the bowel.

೨3) Drink lots of vegetable broth which is high in potassium and natural minerals to replace fluid and mineral loss. Broth can be made from celery, zucchini, beets, carrots, beet greens, or chard; be careful to avoid the sulphur-containing vegetables such as broccoli, onions and cabbage because of their strong taste. This broth can be seasoned and taken throughout the day.

೨4) The intestinal flora must be replaced with good bacteria such as *acidophilus*.

೨5) One product that absorbs toxicity is *bentonite*. It is a liquid clay with a very large surface area; take 1 tablespoon three times a day.

೨6) Also the powder or capsule form of *psyllium seed* can be taken to absorb the liquid contents from the intestines and bulk the stool. This is taken 1 teaspoon shaken in a jar of water or 2 capsules twice a day taken with only a small amount of water.

Diarrhea can start with food poisoning or an infection and the mechanism of the bowel is to flush out the irritants with diarrhea. So diarrhea, in fact, may be a beneficial elimination of the infection. It is best not to medicate it to a halt for 24 to 36 hours. The advice given here will make sure it runs its course but is not prolonged. If the diet is not optimum or includes a lot of dairy and acidic fruit, the condition can be prolonged. If the person has an irritable bowel already, or if the bowel is subject to stress, the condition can be prolonged and can sometimes lead to intense investigation that may be worse than the condition.

Some people, after antibiotic therapy, develop diarrhea episodes that may be very difficult to control. The treatment for this form of diarrhea is a yeast-free diet and the use of *acidophilus* to replace the good bacteria. In some cases, testing will have to be performed for yeast in the stool and blood. Candida antibody levels may be checked to determine the extent of the Candida and the appropriate antifungal medication to be given. Please refer to the chapter on **Candidiasis** for further information regarding this condition. If strong medications are needed to treat the diarrhea, remember to follow up with *acidophilus* and an excellent diet so that the medication will not leave an imbalance of the intestinal flora.

Digestive Disorders

༄ A person may eat an optimum diet but there is still the question of proper digestion and absorption of those foods. As we learn more and more about the various digestive processes and how they can go wrong, we are better able to educate people on these conditions. The most important factor in digestion is proper food selection. The second most important aspect is proper food chewing. If a person chews each mouthful of food thirty to forty times, this stimulates the salivary amylase in the mouth and one-third of the digestion can be done in the mouth. If you hold a cooked grain in your mouth long enough, it will become sweet. This is the action of the amylase in breaking down the carbohydrate into glucose.

The action of chewing also stimulates stomach acid production. If a person is under stress or is generally tense, the stomach muscle, like any other body muscle, can be in spasm. This spasm can cut off the circulation of the stomach and decrease production of hydrochloric acid. This reduction in stomach acid can lead to improper or incomplete breakdown of stomach contents, especially protein. If this incompletely digested food finds its way into the intestines by being pushed through in bulk before it is completely digested, then the intestinal flora will feed on this food and create gas and bloating. Incomplete protein digestion can be diagnosed by a urine test called urine indicin.

The third most important aspect of digestion is avoiding water with a meal. Washing down each bite with water dilutes the gastric acid and leads to incomplete digestion, washing food out of the stomach too soon. It also causes the fats and oils in the food to cling together which impedes their absorption. You may drink water 10 minutes before or three hours after eating.

After the stomach, the food passes into the small intestine where bicarbonates neutralize the pH and allow pancreatic amylase to further break down carbohydrates. Also, bile is excreted into the small intestine to emulsify fats. If there is insufficient amylase, carbohydrates will provide food for microorganisms. They can also become fermented in the intestine to the point that alcohol and aldehydes are produced which, in the extreme case, may cause someone to appear drunk. If the fats are not absorbed, the stool is bulky and floats.

In the treatment of digestive disorders, one important thing to look for is chronic stomach spasm or hiatus hernia. The stomach lies central and to the right of the abdomen directly under the sternum which joins the ribs. If that area is hard and painful, it may be that the stomach is in spasm. The stomach can push up between the diaphragm and even restrict the movement of the diaphragm leading to shortness of breath or inability to take a deep breath. The pain can travel around to the back and up the front of the chest. Often times, there is a reflux of acid up the esophagus because the normal sphincter between the esophagus and the stomach is stretched. The treatment for this condition is a type of traction massage on the stomach to relax the stomach and pull it down into its proper position. Many children have this condition after vomiting. Adults who do too many situps get it, women during pregnancy are susceptible, as are people with constipation who are putting more pressure on the stomach. Generalized tension in which the breathing is high in the lungs and the person is afraid or in a constant state of fight of flight can cause the stomach to be "hiked up."

The advice to treat or avoid hiatus hernia or stomach spasms includes:

1. Avoid coffee, tea, and alcohol which relax the sphincter between the stomach and esophagus.
2. Avoid sit-ups or do modified sit-ups.
3. Do not lie down after a meal.
4. Do not drink a lot of liquids with meals.
5. In the morning, to settle the stomach in proper position, drink a glass of water and rise up on your toes then thump down on your heels about ten times.
6. Have a professional massage your stomach hard and down and to the right to try to release the spasm; often you will hear a gurgle as stomach contents that have been trapped are released.

In order to treat digestive disorders, chew the food well, eat when calm, drink no more than four ounces of liquid at each meal so that the gastric juices are not diluted, and eat an optimum diet. If food allergies are suspected, follow the advice in the chapter on **Allergies** regarding food avoidance and challenging or obtain the food allergy tests. Candidiasis can also cause a lot of gastrointestinal upset. Read Dr. Trowbridge's book *The Yeast Syndrome* or Dr. Crook's book *The Yeast Connection*, and refer to the chapter on **Candidiasis**.

Homeopathic remedies for digestive disorders include *Nux vomica* and *Lycopodium*; these can be used in the 6c potency but should be prescribed by a homeopath if they are to be used for a long period of time. Herbal remedies include *Swedish Bitters* and the *mint* teas. Gas with a foul odor is relieved somewhat by taking *charcoal tablets*. This substance absorbs toxins in the intestines and they are eliminated from the body.

Diverticulosis

∾ Diverticulosis, a disease of the large intestine that is a direct result of a refined food diet with a lack of fiber, is becoming almost epidemic in so-called civilized countries. Fiber is extremely important in the large intestine because it provides the bulk against which the muscles of the intestine push out the waste products of digestion. If there is not enough bulk or fiber in the intestines, the areas between the muscles start to form tiny pouches, or sacks, which are called diverticuli, along the outside walls of the large intestine. When there is a lack of fiber in the large intestine, the liquid matter of the intestinal contents tends to be more completely absorbed back into the body; thus the fecal matter becomes drier and harder. As the muscles of the large intestine try to force the hard material along and out the anus, they have to exert more and more muscular force to do this. With all this excess pressure (and often ineffective pressure), constipation results and, with time, the areas between the muscles become like pouches or sacks bulging out the whole length of the intestinal wall. The diagnosis can be made on barium enema x-ray. A small percentage of people with diverticulosis can get an inflammation leading to lower abdominal pain of one of these little diverticuli. This is called diverticulitis. The best way to treat both of these conditions is prevention. Obviously, the first treatment is fiber. Dr. Dennis Burkitt, the "grandfather of fiber," has proved over and over again that people in countries where a high-fiber diet is maintained do not suffer conditions such as diverticulosis. The types of fiber that are available are bran fiber, oat fiber, rice fiber. Of course, vegetables and fruits have a high fiber content, as well as a high water content. When you take fiber, you must increase your liquid intake—6 to 8 glasses of water per day is the usual recommendation. If the food fibers are difficult to tolerate, or if you need extra fiber outside of the diet, psyllium seed powder or capsules are available. Once again, make sure the liquid intake is sufficient. Some people have actually made themselves more constipated by not taking enough liquid with the psyllium. Beans, barley, and legumes are excellent sources of fiber. When you use these foods, be sure to soak them replacing the water several times over 24 hours to reduce their gas-forming ability. People with diverticulosis, and especially diverticulitis, have a lot of problems with gas pains, which leads me to the general diet for diverticulosis.

Avoid processed foods and concentrate on high fiber foods. Watch out for gas-forming foods. Check your tolerance for dairy products, and even whole-wheat, to which many people are allergic or sensitive. The way to do that is to avoid the food for a couple of weeks and then reintroduce it back into your diet. Check the chapters on **Digestion** and **Food Allergies** for more information on these topics.

Seeds, nuts, and popcorn can be a problem for people with diverticulosis, especially if they are not chewed well. Most people do not realize they should be chewing 30 times per bite to make sure food is completely broken down before it gets to the stomach. Do not smoke or drink and avoid caffeine. Exercise is also very important, as it stimulates the muscles of the intestines, and eases bowel movements. See the chapter on **Constipation** for more information.

Dizziness

᪂ When people have a flu or cold, they can feel dizzy. If their blood sugar is low, or if there is a lack of circulation to the inner ear, it can lead to dizziness. The first two conditions can be ruled out by examining the ear canal or ear drum, taking a history for a cold or flu, doing blood sugar tests and making sure the diet is optimum to avoid low blood sugar. Dizziness due to circulation to the inner ear being cut off should be investigated by an ear, nose, and throat specialist, a neurologist, or a vascular specialist. In older age groups, arteriosclerosis can cause hardening of the arteries and cut the circulation to the brain which leads to dizziness. Read the chapter on **Arteriosclerosis**.

Once all these conditions are ruled out and the dizziness still persists, the treatment for suspected eustachian tube block is avoidance of mucus-forming foods such as sugar, dairy and wheat and using teas such as *fenugreek* which thins the mucus; this is taken 1 teaspoon to a cup of boiling water steeped for five to seven minutes. A homeopathic remedy called *Kali mur.* 6c, 4 drops three times a day can be used for eustachian tube blockage. For dizziness itself, *Bryonia* can be used 6c 4 drops three times a day.

Dry Skin

౻ Most people think that dry skin can be treated by external cream applications. However, attention to the diet and what is taken orally is probably more important. The orally taken essential oils such as *evening primrose oil* and *fish oils* in amounts of 3-4 capsules a day are very important. *Cod liver oil* can be taken in liquid form, 1 teaspoon daily. *Zinc* supplementation of 25 mg a day can be very important for skin, hair, and nails. This is in addition to a good general *multiple vitamin and mineral*. In terms of skin care, some people feel that too many showers and baths can strip the normal acid mantle of the skin and allow dehydration and drying of the skin. This can be treated by putting a few tablespoons of apple cider vinegar in the bath and by using neutral pH skin creams.

Drinking enough water is very important. However, do not take water with a meal up to 10 minutes before or three hours after. Water and oil together in the stomach make the oil globules stick together which impedes its absorption.

Dyslexia

(See **Hyperactivity**)

Earaches

꿍 Earaches can be a very frightening condition especially in children because the pain can be intense. Because ear infections can be so dramatic and people are afraid of ear drum damage, they are often treated with antibiotics. Ear infections develop behind the eardrum often from a mucus fluid build-up in which the bacteria may overgrow and begin to cause pressure and inflammation. For any ear pain or suspicion of an ear infection, a doctor should be consulted.

Not all earaches are due to bacteria. Some people feel that recurrent ear infections are due to food allergies. Often avoiding milk, peanut butter and orange juice, as the main culprits, can diminish or stop the infections.

I will quote Michael S. Schmidt from his book *Childhood Ear Infections*. The back cover reads:

"Ear infections are the number one reason parents take their child to a doctor. Many infants and children experience recurrent ear infections despite continual treatment with antibiotics and antihistamines. Lack of response often leads to surgery. Michael Schmidt cites evidence from the most respected medical and scientific journals that conventional drug and surgical treatments for ear infections are overused and often ineffective. Nutritional strategies, allergy management, acupressure, homeopathic medicine, and herbal remedies can build up a child's immune system, heal ear infections, and prevent their recurrence."

Schmidt's complete list of allergens to avoid include dairy products, wheat, eggs, chocolate, citrus, corn, soy, peanuts, shellfish, sugar and yeast. What's left? Lamb, rice, squash, carrots, potatoes, chicken and applesauce. After being on this diet for three weeks, one food may be introduced at a time. That one food should be eaten several times in one day along with the allowed foods. If there is an allergy, it shows up with obvious symptoms.

Local treatments while waiting for the doctor to arrive can have a wide range. Some books suggest that in infants, putting breast milk into the ear can give relief. Herbal remedies are dilute *mullein oil* or *oil of cajeput* or *tea tree oil*. All these oils would be used 1 part oil to 3 parts safflower oil and dropped into the ear. Heel Biotherapeutics also has a liquid formula that can be used in the ear. Of course if there is an ear discharge, drops should not be used until a doctor is consulted.

Homeopathic remedies are dependent on the symptoms. A red hot throbbing ear would call for *Belladonna*. Earache in a fussy irritable child would suggest *Chamomilla*. A splinter-like earache from the throat into the ear would be *Hepar sulph*. The dosage for each would be 6c or 30c using 4 drops every half-hour until the condition subsides. The best advice would be to read the section on **Remedies** in this book and obtain a small homeopathic book such as *Homeopathy at Home* by Dr. Trevor Smith, to have on hand for emergencies. It is important to have a homeopathic first aid kit available to use until you can get to the doctor. Michael Schmidt's book also contains an excellent section on homeopathic remedies. He includes *Aconite, Belladonna, Chamomilla, Ferrum phos., Hepar sulph., Lycopodium, Mercurius, Plantago, Pulsatilla* and *Silica*. Most of these medicines are listed in the second section of this book. A quick read can give you an idea of which symptoms and thus which remedy would fit your child.

Eczema

⤳ Eczema denotes a chronic skin condition that can range from wet blisters to dry flakes and that is usually itchy and can occur on any surface of the body. It is most commonly associated with allergies either by contact or by ingestion and is usually aggravated by stress. One first must trace down the allergic factor by avoiding and challenging certain foods. One might also investigate and treat Candidiasis which can cause or aggravate any skin condition. Once the offending substance is removed, then the skin should normalize.

Most eczemas are dry. The best treatment is to lubricate the body with *cod liver oil*. Don't put it on your skin; take it internally, 1 tablespoon per day. Take it away from water so it will be absorbed and avoid water with the meal so that the fats and oils in foods will be absorbed properly. Water in the stomach simultaneously with oil will cause the oil globules to combine together in an oil puddle which the body will have trouble absorbing.

Avoid showers since they strip the acid mantle of the skin. Use ¼ cup apple cider vinegar, a few drops of bath oil, and a cotton pouch of oatmeal in the bath. Clay is also helpful in a bath to treat eczemas. Dry indoor air is bad for eczema; use a humidifier and use external creams and lotions. Avoid wools and use cottons. Make sure the soap you use does not irritate the skin. Do several rinses on your wash and don't use scented antistatic products in the dryer.

The vitamins and minerals that aid the health of the skin are *evening primrose oil*, 3 to 4 capsules a day; *marine lipids* or *fish oils* 3 to 4 capsules a day; 25 mg a day of *chelated zinc* or *zinc picolinate*. This is in addition to a *multiple vitamin* and *mineral* containing *vitamin A* and the *B vitamins*.

Using cortisone creams for eczema does help the symptoms by suppressing them. However, there is a concern that if an eczema is suppressed the child will later develop other manifestations of allergies such as asthma. Therefore in the beginning of a skin condition, it is important to determine the cause and treat the cause.

There are many homeopathic remedies to treat skin such as *Sulphur* for burning, red, itchy, unhealthy looking skin; *Graphites* for oozy, crusty types; *Petroleum* for dry, cracked, rough skin; or *Mezereum* for painful, small bumpy eczema not on the face. However, these remedies should be properly studied and researched before using. If they do not work after a short time, a homeopath or naturopath should be consulted. Often if cortisones have been used for a long time, the skin may go through an aggravation or worsening before getting better. (Read the chapters on **Allergies** and **Candidiasis**.)

Edema

༄ Edema is a buildup of fluid underneath the skin with an excess of fluid in the interstitial spaces between cells. This area normally holds fluid as it travels between the cells and the lymphatic circulation. The lymph is an extremely important system that carries all the liquid waste product away from the cells, runs it through the body and deposits it in the *cisterna chylae* underneath the right upper ribs. From there, the wastes go into the blood stream and then are excreted usually through the kidneys into the urine or through the skin or the bowels. If the lymphatic system is overloaded or clogged with too many wastes, then edema can build. In very old people, who have very swollen ankles, this is a condition of edema. With age and gravity, the lymph system is completely broken down and fluid falls to the feet.

The lymphatic circulation depends entirely on exercise and movement in order to pump the lymph up to the chest. Methods for improving circulation are dry skin brushing from the feet up to the chest, from the tips of the fingers up the arms to the chest, from the abdomen up to the chest. The motion is brisk and light. There are specialists who do lymphatic massage. It is a very delicate massage which consists of light brushing of the skin in the direction of the flow of the lymph.

Edema in women most often occurs before the menstrual period as the hormones retain more fluid. This can be diminished somewhat by avoiding salt and sugar which also retain fluid in the body. The herbs that will give diuretic effects are *parsley, watermelon seeds, uva ursi* and *nettles*. These can be taken in herbal team form. The formula would be 1 teaspoon per cup steeped for at least ten minutes. A large amount can be made at once and reheated or taken at room temperature. *Vitamin B6* in dosages from 100 to 300 mg per day a week before the period will also act as a natural diuretic. (Read the chapter on **Premenstrual Syndrome** in this book.)

Emphysema

ᑲ This condition can only be treated by prevention. In short, no smoking. Smoking creates a breakdown of the structure of the lung in the alveolar areas; destruction of alveoli leads to empty spaces in the lungs so air exchange can no longer occur. The treatment once this condition has occurred includes avoidance of allergies. Stay away from strong smells and scents. Exercise is important, especially walking and swimming.

The shallow fast breathing of emphysema may create a pulling up of the stomach creating a stomach spasm or hiatus hernia. Learn yogic breathing; when you inhale, let your abdomen rise so your diaphragm falls. This opens up the lungs to full capacity and massages the stomach in place.

Don't eat large meals. This puts pressure on the diaphragm. Eat small frequent meals and try to keep to an optimum body weight.

Most communities have lung rehabilitation facilities to perform physiotherapy and to teach people exercises for the lungs and demonstrate the use of oxygen in the home.

Oxygenating vitamins and minerals could be used; e.g., *vitamin E*, 400 to 800 I.U. per day; *selenium*, 200 mcg per day; *evening primrose oil*, 3 to 4 per day; *beta carotene* 20,000 I.U.; vitamin A, 10,000 I.U. Check with your doctor regarding supplementation. Various algae products have been getting a lot of attention lately. These nutrients are good oxygenators, high in nutrients, and readily absorbed.

Endometriosis

๛ Endometriosis is on the increase. In this condition, the endometrial tissue which lines the uterus is also growing abnormally outside the uterus in the pelvic cavity. It can be growing along the bowel, on the ovaries, along the Fallopian tubes, or around the ligaments that hold up the uterus. Every month, when a woman normally has her period, this endometrial tissue will also swell and bleed, but this blood has nowhere to go, and it can stay in the pelvic cavity and cause a buildup of inflammation and scarring. The symptoms are extremely painful periods, low-back pain, painful bowel movements, and pain on intercourse.

There are many theories as to why endometriosis is occurring. One important finding is that tampon use is a possible contributor to this condition. It is advisable to use sanitary napkins instead. There is at least one brand out now called Stayfree Ultrathin that uses a natural moss in the napkin, which is highly absorptive, very thin and diminishes odor.

Endometriosis may also be an immune system deficiency. Actually, most women have some endometrial tissue growing in the wrong place; yet when the abnormally placed endometrial tissue bleeds, their immune system is able to remove the debris quickly, and there is no accumulation, build-up, or scarring. This may be true of fibrocystic breast disease as well.

Therefore, the main focus of treatment should be to boost

the immune system and its ability to clear away this debris. Dietary advice is to avoid caffeine, alcohol, and sugar, and to eat an optimum diet of vegetables, fruit, whole grains, nuts, seeds, legumes, fish and chicken. Fish is especially important for its fish oil, which has an anti-inflammatory property.

Menstrual pain can be treated medically with anti-prostaglandin agents, drugs that suppress the prostaglandins that create cramping. But natural prostaglandins, such as *fish oils*, are important, and prostaglandins that reduce cramping are also available in the form of *evening primrose oil*. This has been researched and proven effective in some clinical trials in the treatment of endometriosis.

Other recommendations are for *calcium and magnesium*, which have natural anti-cramping properties; *vitamin E*, which is also useful in endometriosis, as well as the *B complex*; along with a good *multiple vitamin and mineral* supplement. The other recommendations include using *castor oil packs*. Castor oil has been proven to enhance lymphatic clearing of toxins. It is used externally; an old hand towel or face cloth or layer of flannel is soaked with castor oil, wrung out and placed over the abdomen, covered with another towel, and finally with a heating pad or hot water bottle. If this treatment is done for at least an hour on a daily basis, there can be a great reduction in the pain. I think this treatment probably helps to stimulate the lymphatic system in the pelvic area to clear away the menstrual discharge that occurs in the pelvis.

I have found that acupuncture helps this condition. This leads me to believe that there must be a degree of energy-blocking in this area which would be worth exploring with a psychotherapist.

Epilepsy

Epilepsy refers to a condition of the brain where the firing of impulses in the brain are disordered due to a focus of scar tissue. The effect on the body can be seen in extension and contraction of the arms and legs as in *grand mal* epilepsy or abnormal movements of the lips, staring of the eyes and loss of time in *petit mal*. Often brain scans find no focus of abnormality yet the symptoms still occur.

Perhaps the person also has an underlying blood sugar abnormality or a vitamin or mineral deficiency. Low blood sugar can cause a decreased supply of glucose to the brain and trigger the epileptic episode at those times. (Read the chapter on **Hypoglycemia** in this book.)

Mineral deficiency has been implicated in epilepsy. *Magnesium, zinc* and *manganese* are three minerals that should be investigated. A hair analysis could be obtained to see if these minerals are deficient.

Some people feel that the muscle contractions of epilepsy continue because the body is unable to burn up the acetylcholine. Inositol and lecithin can be used to balance choline. The alkaline B vitamins would be more important than the acid B vitamins. The alkaline B's are *inositol* and *lecithin*. The acid B's are *B13, B15, B17* and *folic acid*. *Taurine*, an amino acid, is being studied for its anti-epileptic properties.

An herbal treatment for epilepsy due to trauma of whiplash with consequent congestion of cerebrospinal fluid is *black cohosh* or *cimicifuga* in tincture form 10 drops in water two or three times a day. Trauma is one of the predisposing factors to epilepsy. Immediately after head injury, *vitamin E*, 400 to 800 units, and *selenium*, 200 mcg should be taken.

The trauma of birth has been implicated in some forms of epilepsy. I consider it very important for parents to have a cranial assessment on their newborn to determine whether the sutures of the skull bones are jammed after a particularly difficult birth. Specialists who do this type of work are called craniosacral massage therapists.

Epstein-Barr

⁓ This condition has been renamed chronic fatigue syndrome (CFS). In Canada and Britain it is called ME, myalgic encephalo-myelitis. This identifies the muscles and brain as the target sites of symptoms. It appears to be a reactivation of an already pres-ent mononucleosis-like virus. Apparently up to 90 percent of the population has antibodies to Epstein-Barr, meaning they have had an infection. To most people, it would seem like a normal cold or flu. With some people, primary infection can be severe like mononucleosis and the person never recovers. Or the reactivation of the virus can be severe and can leave the person feeling fatigued, run down and "never well since" that time.

The symptoms are chronic headaches, swollen glands, peri-odic fevers and chills, muscle aches and pains, muscle weakness, sore throat and numbness and tingling of extremities. The gen-eral feeling is one of incredible fatigue and inability to do even the simplest of tasks plus an inability to cope with any stress. The cognitive dysfunction seems to be the worst part. People cannot write or do math or remember. Pain is another key to diagnosis. Pain anywhere in the body can lead to multiple inves-tigations and even surgeries in search of the elusive cause.

I consider CFS to be a new presentation of an old virus which to me means that the population that is getting this virus is more run down and stressed. They have had a reactivation of the virus because their body was not strong enough to fight it off or they came in contact with a chemical or pollutant that undermined their resistance and allowed them to succumb to the illness. The typical person who is diagnosed with CFS is an overworked woman, 30 to 50 years of age who works with the public as a nurse or teacher. She was recently immunized, trav-eled abroad, and/or has taken a lot of antibiotics over the years, possibly developing candidiasis on top of CFS.

There is no specific treatment for EBV (or CFS) but I suggest plenty of vegetables, gentle exercise, rest and various natural supplements such as the *B vitamins, magnesium, vitamin C* and a *multiple vitamin. Evening primrose oil* in the form of Efamol with *cod liver oil* or *fish oils* seems to be the treatment that works best for this condition. I would also add *echinacea*, an herbal-antibiotic that can be taken on a regular basis to avoid reinfection as well as *B12* shots to increase the energy level. B12 has the ability to strengthen the nervous system. There may be homeopathic remedies that help some people but if the vital force is very low, homeopathic remedies might create an aggravation of the existing condition so they should be used with much caution.

Eyes

One of the highest concentrations of vitamin C in the body is found in the vitreous part of the eye. Good eye health depends on the general health of the individual.

Red eyes can be infected or allergic. If they're infected with a bacteria, the discharge tends to be yellow and sticky and the eyes are itchy and sometimes painful. At this point, the treatment may require a sulpha or antibiotic eyedrop. If it is a viral infection, the discharge may be more watery. A painful eye can even be a herpes infection with a blister in the eye. A doctor must use a special light called a slit lamp to check for a herpes blister on the eye or a scratch or abrasion that has become infected. The eye might have to be treated with an antibiotic cream and patched overnight to heal the abrasion and prevent bacterial infection in the abrasion.

If allergic, the treatment is with particular herbal or homeopathic eye rinses or drops. These are available in most health food stores. One such herb is *eyebright* or *euphrasia*. Sometimes a mild eye infection can respond to these herbs as well. You can puncture a capsule of *vitamin A oil* and drip the contents into the open eye for any sort of eye infection. But, of course, check with your doctor first.

Tired over-worked eyes can then be rested with (used or weak) *chamomile tea*-bags. Put them on while warm. People with sensitive eyes should avoid the chlorine in swimming pools.

Fatigue

꙳ One of the most frequent complaints brought to doctors by their patients is fatigue. The causes of fatigue are multiple and can include allergies, anemia—whether from iron, copper or B12 deficiency, Epstein-Barr, recurrent mononucleosis, hepatitis, hypothyroidism, or Candidiasis. All of the above can be diagnosed with various clinical tests. Also read the indicated chapters in this book. Other conditions include depression, insomnia and stress. The fatigue can lead to lack of exercise which perpetuates the vicious cycle because exercise can banish some forms of fatigue. A person should not be content with anything less than optimal health and should strive to obtain this with an excellent diet, good sleep habits and, of course, regular exercise. The above conditions should be researched and investigated with the doctor in order to determine the cause of the fatigue.

Fever

(SEE BABY TIPS)

Fibrocystic Breast Disease

꙳ This is an increasingly common condition in women. The factors that are cited for fibrous tissue in the breasts are: salt, a high protein diet, too much meat and dairy, and the theobromine substances in coffee, tea and chocolate. A lot of people have heard that avoidance of coffee will help diminish breast lumps or pain. It is not the caffeine that is responsible here but the theobromines. This condition does not lead to breast cancer but is important to treat because fibrous tissue in the breast can mask developing breast cancer. The best treatment is prevention by avoiding these foods.

A diet high in whole grains, vegetables, and beans and low in fat helps excrete estrogen, which means less estrogen to stimulate the breasts. Such a diet will help with weight loss as well. Overweight women have too much estrogen which can stimulate the breasts. Women on the birth control pill can be affected by the daily estrogen stimulation and may have to find another form of birth control.

Oral iodine supplementation in a natural form may be helpful. Dr. William Ghent of the Hotel Dieu Hospital in Kingston, Ontario has been researching fibrocystic breast disease and iodine for many years. His work, published in the *Canadian Journal of Surgery* (October 1993), shows that more than 80 percent of the women he has seen can be markedly helped by the intake of iodine.

Other nutrients that have been used for this condition are *evening primrose oil*, 4 to 6 capsules a day and *vitamin E*, 400 I.U.'s a day. *Vitamin B6*, 50 to 200 mg per day is helpful, especially taken before the period when breasts swell due to stimulation by the rising female hormones. The treatment of **Premenstrual Tension** and **Candidiasis** are also important in the treatment of painful fibrocystic breast disease. Please read these chapters.

Fibroids

෴ Fibroids are a benign overgrowth of the muscles in the wall of the uterus. This is not a pre-cancerous condition. It can lead to stretching of the uterus lining which can cause heavier bleeding and more cramping during the period. The medical treatment is a hysterectomy if the symptoms of bleeding or pain are debilitating. There is always a controversy around the removal of fibroids and it does seem to depend on the particular specialist's approach.

The treatment up to the point of surgery is difficult to delineate because there is very little research on the treatment of fibroids. Some people feel that a low saturated fat diet such as Nathan Pritikin proposed for heart disease would be beneficial. Also the intake of unsaturated fatty acids such as *evening primrose oil*, 4 capsules per day and *marine lipid* capsules, 4 per day as well as *vitamin E*, 400 units per day and *vitamin A*, 20,000 units per day is recommended. These are taken in conjunction with a good *multiple vitamin and mineral*. Foot reflexology massage has helped diminish the pain from fibroids and in some cases even diminished the fibroid itself. External castor oil packs can help the pain and congestion created by the fibroids.

If the condition does become debilitating, find a doctor who is willing to consider removing the fibroid alone without the removal of the uterus. This can be done with very large fibroids which are in a good position to be removed and the woman may even become pregnant thereafter. An excellent book on this topic is *No More Hysterectomies* by Dr. Vicki Hufnagel.

First Aid

&. The most effective first aid I know is with the use of homeopathy and herbal remedies. A good manual is Dr. Dorothy Shepperd's *Homeopathy for the First Aider*. For a quick rundown of conditions and treatments:

&.1. For **pain, aching, bruising** (from dental extractions, sprains of joints, fractured bones and concussions), *Arnica* is given either 6c or 30c by mouth every two hours. Arnica can be used in tincture or cream form locally for contusions, bruising or swelling. However, if the skin is broken at all Arnica is inappropriate for topical application and must not be used. Calendula tincture is then used and is also a good antiseptic.

∽2. **For stabs, puncture wounds, bites, stings or splinters,** oral *Ledum* is used 6c every one-half to four hours repeated when the pain returns. Ledum tincture or calendula tincture can be used topically.

∽3. **For puncture wounds, injury to coccyx or spinal concussion,** oral *Hypericum* is used, 6 or 30c, 4 drops every two to four hours. Hypericum can also be used for crushed fingers or toes or any abrasion where nerve endings are irritated, such as abrasion of the palm of the hand or the knee. In these abrasions, Hypericum tincture can be used on the surface of the skin. Hypericum can also be used for the phantom pain of an amputated limb.

∽4. **For sprained tendons or ligaments** or bruised bone or inflammation of ligaments or joints, or bruises of the shin, *Ruta* is especially useful (after Arnica 6c) 6c 4 drops every one to four hours as needed. It is also good for eye injuries.

∽5. **For the healing of fractures** of the bone, oral *Symphytum* 6 or 30c is extremely useful for speedy healing.

∽6. **For ruptured ligaments and tendons** around joints, especially wrists and ankles, *Rhus tox.* is the best remedy, 6 to 30c, 4 drops every two to four hours.

∽7. **For wounds,** *Calendula* or *Hypericum* tincture can be put in water to clean and wrap a wound; they both have antiseptic as well as analgesic properties. They can also stop a local hemorrhage.

∽8. **For hemorrhaging,** *Calendula* tincture can be applied directly. For dental hemorrhage, oral *Phosphorus* 6 or 30c every ten to fifteen minutes will stop the bleeding. For nosebleeds,

Ferrum phos. 6c or *Vipera* 6c every fifteen minutes will stop bleeding.

🕮9. **For burns and scalds,** apply cold water immediately. *Urtica urens* by mouth, 6 or 30c, and locally in a tincture will help the pain. In severe cases with great pain and restlessness, *Causticum* by mouth, 30 or 200c, and *Hypericum* tincture externally is used. The most severe burns are treated with oral *Cantharis,* 30c or 200c.

Flat Feet

🕮 One has flat feet when the arch of the foot loses its elevation and touches the floor. People who have this condition can be miserable with chronically sore and achy feet. You can diagnose yourself by stepping out of a pool or tub onto a surface which will show the outline of your sole. If the whole foot imprint shows, then you have flat feet. An elevated arch will not touch and wet the surface at all.

Flat feet seem to be hereditary and it is possible that they can't be avoided. However, if children grew up wearing proper shoes with proper supports, the arch might be maintained. Sneakers with arch supports can help maintain good foot structure.

Podiatrists and some chiropractors offer orthotic devices to help people with fallen arches or flat feet. These are leather or plastic inserts that are placed in the shoe and are usually constructed from a mold of your foot. They are quite expensive, but some insurance companies cover them and for some people they are indispensable.

Gall Bladder Disease

🕮 The gall bladder stores and concentrates bile that is used to emulsify fats. There is an intricate balance between cholesterol, lecithin and bile acids in the production of bile. If the diet is high in saturated fats, then those fats which are liquid at 149 degrees and solid below that temperature will clog the bile flow and can lead to a build up of cholesterol and subsequent stone formation in the gall bladder. If there is insufficient lecithin, gall stones can also form. The pain from gall bladder attacks is from sludge or stones in the gall bladder that are trying to exit through the narrow bile duct under the stimulation of fat in the stomach. A fatty meal will stimulate the gall bladder to try to excrete bile for digestion of the fat but will only cause pain. This is the cause of gall bladder attacks.

Another interesting avenue of research is the allergic component of gall bladder attacks. There are many people who have had gall bladder surgery but continue to have pain. Dr. Jonathan Wright's *Guide to Healing with Nutrition* has a chapter on foods which have been shown to stimulate gall bladder pain. Other than medications, the biggest offenders were eggs, pork, onions, fowl, milk, coffee and oranges. It would be useful to explore this avenue before attempting surgical intervention. The treatment for gall bladder problems also includes avoiding all animal fats and attempting a more vegetarian diet.

There are many herbal remedies for the liver and gall bladder that can be taken in tea or tincture form. These include herbs such as *burdock, parsley, garlic, onion, black Russian radish* and *horseradish. Vitamin E,* 400 I.U., *copper* 2 mg, *taurine* 250 mg, and *lecithin,* 1200 mg are also advised by some doctors. A diagnosis of stones can be made by having a gall bladder ultrasound. If there are no stones, a gall bladder flush with a drink that mixes olive oil and lemon juice might be helpful.

Gas

ᕦ It's something we all have, some in more abundance than others. In some people, gas results in belching, and in others it causes flatulence. Flatulence can occur due to lactose intolerance or as a result of eating various foods that are high in the production of gas, such as the cruciferous vegetables (broccoli, Brussels sprouts, cabbage and cauliflower), onions, dried legumes or wheat products. Sometimes it occurs because of improper digestion, ranging from improper chewing to lack of hydrochloric acid in the stomach, to drinking too much water with a meal and allowing incompletely digested food into the intestines where gas-producing bacteria have a field day.

If you lack the enzyme that digests the lactose in milk, there are Lactaid enzymes which you can put in your milk or take after eating dairy products to help you digest this food. Beans and legumes can be soaked 24 hours, removing the water and replacing it several times to reduce the gas-forming substances. Beano is a product which also provides a missing enzyme and can be added to the first mouthful of a bean dish. If there are foods that you are allergic to or sensitive to, these should be avoided. Eliminate suspected foods from the diet and then reintroduce them; see if flatulence returns to determine the foods you should avoid.

More fiber introduced into the diet for health reasons can actually promote gas. It is usually because the body is not used to it, and it may set up a gas in the beginning, so the lesson here is to go slowly when introducing fiber.

Treatment is with various products such as *acidophilus* bacteria. This is the good bacteria in the intestines, and presumably if there is a proper amount of the good bacteria, then the gas-forming bacteria won't have as much chance to form gas. Activated charcoal tablets absorb gases in the intestines and may be a symptomatic treatment for the problem. Bentonite clay, as well, is a symptomatic absorber of gas. Again, gas is just a symptom of a possible imbalance, so instead of using a remedy for the symptom, try to get to the root of the problem and cure the problem entirely. Also read the chapter on **Digestive Disorders**.

Gout

꤯ In gout uric acid builds up usually in the big toe. Gout responds to a low purine diet. It has long been thought that gout is due to a high intake of heavy protein foods. Foods to avoid are coffee, tea, alcohol, chocolate, cocoa, wheat germ, pastries, cookies, cream, cakes, beef, lamb, pork and all fried meat, fried potato and potato chips, bouillon, consomme, meat stock, soups, gravy and yeast. If this diet is strictly adhered to, the incidents of gouty attacks diminish greatly.

Soak the foot in Epsom salts and clay. Put a clay pack on the affected area to draw out the inflammation. Use ice, not heat for relief and keep the foot elevated. Take lots of water to flush out the uric acid.

The supplements that can help are cherry juice taken daily, *folic acid*, 5 mg daily, and *B12* injections. The latter two supplements are given after B12 and folic acid blood tests are performed to insure that the taking of these supplements will not mask an underlying condition of B12 deficiency called pernicious anemia.

Gum Disease

ॐ Gum disease, or gingivitis, may be the result of inadequate dental care. The teeth will build up plaque or tartar, another name for the food debris which coats the teeth. This food debris then becomes a breeding ground for organisms. The usual organisms are thought to be bacteria, and the common advice for dealing with this plaque and tartar is to brush and floss your teeth properly. The plaque can also occur at the gum line and cause irritation of the gums, leading to bleeding and infection of the gum line, or pyorrhea.

The correct way to brush is at a 45 degree angle at the gum line, using small side-to-side motions down the teeth, so that the gum and the tooth are both taken care of. Rinsing with half water, half 3 percent hydrogen peroxide to remove bacteria from the mouth is also advised. Baking soda will change the pH of the mouth and allow a less hospitable environment for bacteria. Eating raw vegetables can certainly help the teeth be-

cause it cleans the teeth and stimulates the gums at the same
time. Some people use oral irrigation units to flush the debris
away from the teeth. Cigarette smoking and alcohol drinking
have a negative effect on the mouth and can also deplete your
body's vitamins and minerals.

Gum disease is thought to be the precursor of osteoporosis
in the jawbones, so calcium-rich foods are recommended: dark
green, leafy vegetables, nuts and seeds, sardines, salmon, and
dairy products, if you're not allergic to them. If you take a
calcium supplement, use it along with a *magnesium* supplement.
Vitamin C and *bioflavinoids* are also recommended; one of the
first signs of scurvy (a deficiency of vitamin C) is bleeding gums.
The bioflavinoids are especially important for capillary healing.

One of the things that is missing in the recommendations
concerning gum disease is the awareness that parasites and yeast
organisms also make their home in the mouth. A coated white
tongue or white patches along the inside of the mouth that
can be removed, indicate an oral thrush. Yeast organisms will
overgrow in a body where the sugar intake is high, in people
who use oral cortisones, cortisone nasal drops, or even cortisone
air-puffers for asthma. It also can occur in people who take
antibiotics.

Many dentists recommend antibiotics prior to teeth cleaning
for those who have mitral valve prolapse. It seems that more
and more people are being diagnosed with these murmurs, probably because of increased technology. It is unfortunate that so
many people are being prescribed antibiotics to prevent the possibility of a very rare infection of the heart valves after dental
work. I cannot advise you to avoid these antibiotics for this
purpose. Each person has to decide for him or herself. However,
where there is a severe allergy to the antibiotics recommended,
patients have used high doses of *echinacea*, 20 drops in 4 ounces
of water, taken four times per day a few days before, and five
days or so after, dental work. (Please read the chapter on **Candidiasis** for more information about the condition of yeast overgrowth that can affect the mucous membranes of the mouth,
just as it can the gastrointestinal tract and the vagina in women.)

I see cases where people have a thick, raw, beefy tongue; bleeding, sore, burning mucous membranes; and indentations along the tongue from the teeth. This condition responds to Candida treatment and high doses of the *B vitamins*. The burning mouth syndrome is often amenable to the B vitamins, but since Candida is often a factor, then the B vitamins should be from a non-yeast source.

Parasites are another class of organism that is often forgotten by dentists and periodontists. These can only be seen by direct microscopy; swabs or saliva from the mouth must be viewed immediately under a microscope to see these organisms. The treatment has to be with an antifungal agent; however, most oral antifungal agents are so harsh that there are many side effects, one of them being an overgrowth of yeast in the body. The most natural remedy for this condition is a new product in the health food stores made from *grapefruit seed extract*, and there are many brands available. This extract is a very viscous liquid, the more thick and viscous, probably the stronger. It is extremely bitter, and sometimes, for intestinal parasites, it can be put in capsules, but for use in the mouth it must be in a water solution, 2 or 3 drops in 3 ounces of water. This must be gargled and rinsed in the mouth for several minutes; you don't need to swallow the solution. If this is done twice a day, the parasites will be taken care of. The health of the whole body will have to be looked at here, because the reason there is gum disease, or gingivitis, could be a deficiency of many vitamins or minerals from an imbalanced diet. An optimum diet should be followed, including a lot of vegetables, with a moderate amount of fruit, nuts, seeds, whole grains, beans, legumes, fish and chicken. Avoid sugar, alcohol, and coffee. Use dairy products if you're not allergic to them. Use the supplements I've mentioned before—*vitamin C, calcium and magnesium, vitamin A* (very important for the mucous membranes) as well as a good *multiple vitamin and mineral.*

Hayfever

(SEE **ALLERGIES**)

Headaches

↬ The most common types of headaches I see are tension, migraine, hypoglycemic, allergic, chronic fatigue and post-motor vehicle accident headaches.

Stress headaches can begin the vicious cycle to tension headaches. Physical or emotional stress can contribute. Physical misuse of the body such as sitting too long at a desk without taking a break can cause cramping and tightening of muscles. Periodic stretching is recommended. Yoga is also an exceptional exercise to help keep the whole body flexible.

Hypoglycemic or low blood sugar headaches are one of the many symptoms of hypoglycemia. (See that chapter for a full discussion). If a meal is skipped and the brain is deprived of glucose, a hypoglycemic individual will feel foggy or dizzy; if the warning signal is not heeded and food is still not taken, a full blown headache can result. Some people get tension headaches and some migraines.

The treatment is obvious. Keep the blood sugar up with small frequent meals and avoid sweets.

Poor sleep position can also lead to neck pain and consequent headaches. Lying on the stomach is especially harmful. Keeping the whole body in alignment is the key. The head should not be propped up on several pillows. There are special neck posture pillows that you can purchase or you might try rolling up a small soft towel and placing that under your neck with the head on a flat pillow. If you lie on your side, the towel should be under your neck as well. Adequate support to the neck, in this way, prevents neck tension and spasm.

Emotional stress is a major cause of headaches. It can occur suddenly or creep up insidiously over time. Most of us have had the experience of receiving some shocking news and immediately the heart races, the adrenaline pours out, the blood rushes to our head and pounds in our ears and a headache is born. Crying only intensifies the pain.

Relief may come with a quick resolution to the situation but, if the stress is ongoing, certain natural measures can be taken.

A cold pack on the forehead, eyes and/or the neck may give symptomatic relief. A hot shower or soothing bath or footbath may calm the whole body, since it is a whole body reaction to stress. A neck and head massage is helpful and also comforting.

Chronic emotional stress can lead to chronic tension headaches which must be treated more aggressively. Tension headaches can occur from a progression of long-standing muscle spasms of the neck and shoulders that over time begin to encroach upon the muscles of the scalp. This causes pulling and strain on the scalp and also can begin to jam the underlying sutures of the cranial bones. Muscle spasms can be extremely powerful to the point of actually breaking or dislocating bones. In the upper back and neck, a muscle spasm can cause rotation of the vertebrae of the neck or a rib dislocation and severe pain. A muscle spasm will have a decreased blood flow in the center of the spasm. The lack of circulation will allow build up of waste products in that area which can lead to scarring and calcification. When a muscle spasm becomes this chronic, it is then referred to as fibrositis.

The treatment for the condition at this point is very deep and painful muscle massage to try to break down the calcification, increase the circulation to the area and return normal function.

Whiplash or other head and neck injuries can lead to the same series and progression of events. Treatment for these types of headaches begins with an optimum diet, adequate rest, gentle stretching exercises, massage and sometimes deep massage for the calcified, scarred areas of the muscles, plus cranial massage if the headaches have begun jamming the cranial bones. (See the chapter on **Epilepsy**.) Chiropractic adjustment is often necessary to release the cervical vertebrae but adequate attention must be paid to the muscle component. It is often the muscles that are in spasm that are pulling the vertebrae out of alignment and frequent adjustments are not going to help if the muscles are still in spasm. Some patients find that chronic neck and back problems after back injury are helped by cleansing programs such as *aloe vera gel*, one tablespoon each morning in juice or water. (See the chapter on **Detoxification**.)

Migraine headaches have a component of light sensitivity, nausea, sometimes vomiting, and these symptoms are felt to be due to the intensity of pain. However, research done in England on migraines shows that up to 85 percent have been made headache-free with the elimination of cigarette smoke, pork, oranges, wheat, eggs, chocolate, dairy, sugar, beef, tea and coffee. It is worthwhile avoiding these possible irritants for a sufficient period of time to determine if they might be creating the migraine situation. Keep a food diary since any food could be the culprit.

Sinus headaches are often quite painful and difficult to diagnose and treat. During a cold, if some of the bacteria take up residence in the sinus cavities, they can cause a swelling of the mucous membranes with a build up of mucus and lots of painful pressure.

If the throbbing pain in the forehead and face is made worse by bending over, that is one clue to diagnosis. There are sinus cavities above the eyes, beside the nose and in the cheekbones. Finger pressure over these areas usually elicits pain.

Treatment of the underlying infection is aimed at draining the sinuses and eliminating the bacteria involved. This will resolve the sinus headache. (See **Sinusitis** for a full discussion.)

Allergic headaches can take many forms. They can be due to inhaling chemicals that cause neurologic pain, or they can irritate the mucus membranes of the respiratory system and cause inflammation and pain.

Food allergies can create waste products that circulate in the brain, also causing spasm and pain. An allergic reaction to yeast and mold is a good example. Their metabolic waste products include aldehydes and alcohol which can cause headaches.

To diagnose allergic headaches, the onset is important. If you only get these headaches in a particular environment or after a particular meal, then you can begin to narrow down the cause and avoid it. Read the chapter on **Allergies** for a more in depth discussion.

A sudden onset of a new type of head pain, not relieved by sleep, causing waking at night or associated with blood from the eyes, nose or ears must be investigated immediately by your doctor.

An herb called *feverfew* is sometimes helpful in alleviating headaches and may be tried 2 to 6 capsules per day, to be taken when the headache occurs.

Feverfew may also act as a preventive. If you have eliminated all possible causes of your headaches but are still suffering, try taking 4 to 6 capsules on a daily basis to see if there is improvement. Do this for a trial period of three to four weeks, but only after consulting with your doctor. *Calcium* and *magnesium* can be used to relax muscles and for pain relief.

Heartburn

Normally, there is a protective sphincter between the esophagus and the stomach. If, for some reason that sphincter is weakened, then acidic stomach contents can be pushed into the esophagus, which can cause burning pain. This is called "heartburn" because the area of pain is close to the heart. Thus people with heartburn are often mis-diagnosed with angina or heart pain. It is a condition that should be taken care of, so that this mis-diagnosis does not occur. The stomach is built to handle a very strong acid, but the esophagus is not. The things that can weaken the sphincter and allow this reflex of acid into the esophagus can include a large meal which contains a lot of spicy, gassy, fermenting-type food. With the extra stretching on the stomach, and especially if one lies down, the stomach contents can then be pushed up into the esophagus.

First of all, never lie down after a meal. The substances that are most apt to relax the sphincter between the esophagus and the stomach are alcohol, coffee, tomatoes, tobacco, and physical factors such as bending forward while lifting (instead of bending at the knees), overdoing sit-ups, or going to bed shortly after eating. Stress can also weaken the sphincter because, under stress, we tend to breathe shallowly; this means that the breathing is not moving the diaphragm in a rhythmic motion that also massages the abdominal contents and keeps the stomach in place.

When we are under stress, the stomach and abdomen tend to get tense, which can lock the diaphragm in place so it can't move with breathing, and the breathing is shallow. This can lead to stomach spasm, which can mimic a hiatus hernia, and can lead to problems with digestion. If you try to eat a big meal, spicy food, or a carbonated beverage when your stomach is in spasm, it will not be able to hold much content, and will start looking for a way out. If, at the same time you're drinking coffee or alcohol, then the sphincter at the esophagus will weaken, and the stomach contents will push up into the esophagus.

Another way that heartburn can begin is after gastroenteritis with nausea and vomiting. When the esophageal sphincter opens up, the esophagus may become irritated or burned from the contents, and the esophageal sphincter can be left weakened. In this case, the gastroenteritis will be followed by stomach spasm and heartburn which is thought to be part of the gastroenteritis. The treatment at this time is to gently massage the stomach from the tip of the xiphoid process which is at the bottom of the sternum (that little space between the ribs where they attach to the sternum or the breastbone). You start massaging from there down along the right-hand side of the ribcage; massaging in one downward movement to the right several times will often take the spasm out of the stomach and direct it back into place. See the chapter on **Digestion** for more information on stomach spasm and hiatus hernia.

To avoid heartburn, the best advice is to avoid the foods and drinks that have been already mentioned. Practicing food-combining would probably be a good idea in order to stop any fermentation process in the stomach. See the chapter on **Food Combining**. The chapter on **Digestion** also discusses proper chewing, etc.

Herbal remedies for soothing the condition are *ginger*, as a tea or in capsule form. Herbs such as *catnip* and *fennel* are also useful for heartburn. *Slippery elm* can help soothe the esophageal sphincter. An old folk remedy prescribes one teaspoon of *apple cider vinegar* in four ounces of water to be taken throughout a meal to help digest the food. I've noticed myself that mint teas seem to make the problem worse, even though there are many after-dinner mints on the market; in fact, mint actually weakens the esophageal sphincter. I do not recommend antacids, although they do coat the esophagus and the stomach and settle the fermentation in the stomach, helping to push things through. However, they interfere with digestion and only offer symptomatic relief; they do not get at the root of the problem.

Heart Disease

(SEE ANGINA PECTORIS)

Heat Exhaustion

༤ Heat exhaustion occurs when body fluids are lost by sweating and not replenished. Salt also can be lost through the skin, it's not just water that comes through. When you think of the surface area the skin covers, you can understand the potential for enormous loss of fluids over a period of time.

I am seeing this condition more often: people are staying out in the sun too long, not drinking enough water, forgetting simple measures such as wearing a hat in the sun and staying out in the direct sun between eleven o'clock and two o'clock. You should have water with you at all times if you're going to be outdoors. Eating more fruits and vegetables is helpful because of their high water content. Salt tablets should be avoided because they take water away from the extremities and bring it to the stomach to dilute the salt in the stomach before the salt can be absorbed and find its way into the bloodstream. The best way to get salt is by eating vegetables that have their own sodium content. High-sugar drinks are counter-productive for the same reason—the sugar has to be diluted in the stomach first. Fruit is a much better way to keep your blood sugar up and to hold on to water. Obviously, you should avoid coffee, alcohol, and smoking: these dehydrate the body and cause blood vessel constriction. Suspect dehydration when urination slows down—or stops.

When heat exhaustion is on its way to heatstroke, there can be headache, neck pain, dizziness, nausea, and disorientation. Certainly, if heatstroke is suspected, the best place to be is in the hospital. Otherwise, a cool, dark room with air-conditioning or fans is sufficient, and cool water can be applied with a spray bottle or cool towels, which is better than total immersion. Water is the best fluid to take in, and the next best is water with lemon and a bit of honey. This replenishes the sodium and sugar. Then vegetable juices or vegetable broth are recommended.

Hemorrhoids

৯. Hemorrhoids occur in the anal canal and are internal or external to the canal. They are weakened, swollen veins that can swell and even bleed due to pressure from the liver's portal circulation, pressure from constipation or straining the abdomen in any way. They cause a fair amount of disability and irritation when they occur.

The treatment is to avoid liver congestion and to eat an optimum diet, avoiding alcohol, cigarettes and drugs. Avoid constipation with a high fiber diet including bran and beets. Foods that help veins to regain elasticity are garlic, onions, lecithin, okra, green leafy vegetables, and whole grains. Use plenty of liquids and avoid straining at stool. Veins in the body are strengthened by using *bioflavins*, which are part of the *vitamin C complex*. These nutrients help treat varicose veins, uterine hemorrhage and strokes. They are taken in tablet form, 500 mg, 1 to 2 a day. Food sources are buckwheat or citrus pulp.

Local treatments are with baking soda to take away the itch, *witch hazel* in a sitz bath and *vitamin E oil* on the area to relieve swelling. To ease swelling and pain, grate a small amount of raw potato and apply or coat a small piece of potato the size of your small finger with vitamin E and insert into the anus. For swelling, bleeding and pain, apply *comfrey ointment*. For pain and to assist shrinking of the swollen tissues, apply *plantain and yarrow ointment*. Homeopathic *Witch hazel* by mouth 6c, 4 drops three times a day is also helpful.

Sitz baths are very helpful. Use one herb or a combination of: witch hazel, plantain leaves, comfrey root or white oak bark. These herbs are all strong astringents. Use 4 oz of dried herb and ½ gallon of boiling water. Steep for 8 hours, strain, pour some into a shallow pan, and sit in it for 15 minutes.

Medical treatment for small hemorrhoids which have an itching, irritating component, is with a cold suppository called *Anurex*, which is inserted into the rectum to decrease the inflammation of small hemorrhoids, fissures or for anusitis (inflammation of the anus). *Zinc ointment* and *vitamin E* are very good for healing fissures. Most of the above suggestions for hemorrhoids are useful for fissures.

With both conditions, pay special attention to cleaning the anus after a bowel movement; tiny sharp particles in the feces can cut the anal skin. A bidet would be the best solution so you could wash the area immediately after a bowel movement. Otherwise use soft, undyed, unscented toilet paper. Wet some paper and try to clean the first inch of the anal canal. A warm wash cloth with neutral pH soap would help.

The surgical treatment can be very simple for single hemorrhoids. A very tight rubber band is placed at the base of the hemorrhoid in order to cut off any circulation; the hemorrhoid is then absorbed or sloughed off.

Hiatus Hernia

(SEE DIGESTION)

Hyperactivity

There is no doubt that some children are more hyper than others. Hyperactivity has many causes including our electric environment, television, fluorescent lighting, chemicals in our water, additives in our foods, not to mention the highly refined diet overloaded with sugar and white flour so many children consume. There may also be a muscular imbalance of the eyes leading to a form of dyslexia or incoordination between the right and left sides of the brain that may result in hyperactive behavior. All these various causes must be investigated for each individual child. There are no easy answers.

The dietary factors are at least within our control. Children should not be given sugar or junk food and the most allergenic foods, such as dairy and wheat, should be avoided to see if the child's behavior changes. Foods with coloring or additives are also suspect. Some children may be deficient in certain vitamins and minerals. If dairy is avoided, *calcium* and *magnesium* should be provided. Some children are deficient in *zinc* which may turn up on a hair analysis.

The various books on hyperactivity by Dr. Ben Feingold or

Dr. Doris Rapp are excellent resources to help you investigate and understand this condition. Also you might have your child assessed by a practitioner of educational kinesiology or "one brain" treatments. The need for brain balancing in your hyperactive or dyslexic child can be determined by finding out if he is using the same dominant eye as hand. If the child is righthanded, have him look at a distant object through a small hole in a piece of paper which will only permit the right eye to see. If the child cannot see through this hole, this may mean there is a lot of extra processing that the brain has to do in order to perform tasks. The same is true for left eye and left hand. The exercise to help balance right and left brain is simple marching with the arms swinging opposite to each leg.

Hypertension

Hypertension means elevated blood pressure. The top reading of blood pressure is called systolic and is the force of blood that pushes out against the blood vessels. The lower reading, called diastolic, is the back pressure on the heart. The diastolic is the more important reading in terms of heart disease. In a healthy person, blood pressure does not rise with age; but in North America it commonly does, reflecting the conditions of hardening of the arteries and weakness of the heart so prevalent in our society. The systolic pressure will become elevated as the arteries harden with cholesterol and calcium deposition. The diastolic will become elevated as the heart and lungs weaken.

Blood pressure can also become elevated due to mineral deficiencies such as magnesium and calcium. Stress and tension are also known causes of hypertension. People can benefit from relaxation exercises as well as physical exercise. The natural treatment for hypertension is weight loss, exercise, low fat diet, *calcium* and *magnesium* along with a good *multiple vitamin* and *mineral*.

If these measures don't bring your blood pressure down, it is very important prior to going on antihypertensive medications to have a 24 hour blood pressure monitor performed. This enables both doctor and patient to understand whether this condition is present at all times or only at times of stress. It will prevent the overuse of medication.

The chapters on **Arteriosclerosis** and **Angina** should be read as these factors also affect the blood pressure.

Hyperventilation

⌘ Hyperventilation is caused by breathing too fast usually because of anxiety. When someone is afraid or anxious, the adrenalin or fight-or-flight mechanisms start taking over. The blood pumps faster, the heart pounds, more anxiety builds and the person starts breathing too quickly. As part of the primitive fight-or-flight reflex, where the person would be running away from something threatening, or fighting somebody, this extra oxygen would be necessary. However, when you're standing still and having an anxiety attack, this rapid breathing can be frightening.

The best treatment is breathing in and out into a paper bag; the carbon dioxide being exhaled and lost during hyperventilation will be absorbed back into your body and will shut down the mechanisms that are perpetuating the rapid breathing. It helps to have someone with you who can coach you to take slower breaths and help you relax.

Things that exaggerate anxiety and hyperventilation are coffee, alcohol, and cigarette smoking. Read the chapter on **Anxieties** for more information on this condition.

Hypoglycemia

⌘ Hypoglycemia means low blood sugar. Medically, it is only recognized if the blood sugar drops below a certain range (50 mg% or 2.7 grams/dl glucose); however, it can vary depending on the individual and the circumstances. Ideally blood sugar should stay within a certain normal range. However, if a person eats a highly refined diet, the blood sugar will quickly become elevated as this food is rapidly absorbed into the blood stream. When the blood sugar reaches a certain maximum, insulin is stimulated to enter the blood stream and take the excess glucose away into the cells of the body. The insulin that is released is dependent upon the rate of increase of the blood sugar. If a great amount of insulin is released, then the blood sugar may fall dramatically. When the blood sugar falls in a precipitous manner, adrenaline is stimulated to make sure the blood sugar does not fall too low, rendering the person unconscious. The adrenaline stimulates the sugar stores (glycogen) but it can also produce a "fight or flight" reaction. A person may feel a sense of anxiety or impending doom for no apparent reason. At this point, if a meal of refined food or a coffee and a donut are taken, the person may feel better quite quickly but the cycle of rapid elevation of blood sugar and then rapid decline repeats itself and such individuals go through life as if on a roller coaster; we call it the "crash and burn syndrome."

It is important to diagnose this condition properly. It can be done with a glucose tolerance test, although there is much controversy about this testing. A person must keep a journal of her symptoms while having a glucose tolerance test. After 12 to 14 hours of fasting, the person is given a sugar drink and blood is taken every hour for five hours to document what happens to the body's blood sugar over a period of time.

The treatment for hypoglycemia is small frequent meals of complex carbohydrates (vegetables, whole grains, seeds, nuts) and protein. There are authors who suggest either one or the other but it is important to balance both protein and complex carbohydrates in the diet. Sweets, refined foods, and alcohol must be avoided. It may be worthwhile to sit down with a nutritional counsellor to devise proper diet management of this condition.

Supplements that are helpful in treating hypoglycemia are *B vitamins*, 50 mg 1 to 2 a day in a non-yeast base, to support the nervous system; a good *multivitamin and mineral*; *pantothenic acid*, a B vitamin which supports the adrenal glands, 500 mg 1 to 3 a day. For people whose adrenal glands are exhausted, *desiccated adrenal* can also be used for a short time, 1 to 2 tablets at mid-morning and mid-afternoon. *Chromium* is a mineral which has been shown to assist glucose tolerance and balance; 200 micrograms per day would be the normal dose.

Hypothyroidism

∞ The thyroid gland is located on either side of the trachea in the neck. It controls the metabolism of the cells of the body. If the thyroid is low or hypo, then the metabolic rate is lowered. A person can become sluggish, fatigued, have difficulty waking up in the morning, be overweight, have coarsening of the hair and skin, be constipated and have more frequent infections, irregularity of periods and poor wound healing. Since these symptoms overlap with many other conditions, it is important to make an accurate diagnosis. Unfortunately, the blood tests for the thyroid tend to be inaccurate and also can miss an early case of low thyroid.

Dr. Broda Barnes has written an excellent book called *Hypothyroidism; The Unsuspected Illness*. Dr. Barnes suggests that basal body temperature can be a way of assessing metabolic rate. He also suggests using *desiccated thyroid* based on the body temperature to try to supply the thyroid gland with the essential building blocks to support its function. Nutritionally, the supplements *tyrosine, B6, zinc*, and *kelp* may be useful in treating thyroid deficiency. The amount of supplements would have to be individualized for each patient.

Medically, doctors wait until the thyroid is very weak and damaged before using replacement thyroid therapy. Then they use synthetic thyroid hormone.

Incontinence

ᔆ Urinary incontinence is the involuntary loss of urine. It is considered by some to be a regular consequence of aging, but this is not so. Women seem more susceptible to this condition, probably because they have had some weakening of their bladder sphincter muscles during childbirth or may have pressure on the bladder from uterine prolapse. Men, as they get older, are susceptible because the prostate at the base of the penis enlarges and puts pressure on the urethra which causes urinary frequency. (Read the chapter on **Prostate Problems.**)

There is much advice that can help this condition, and one does not have to run out and buy incontinence pads right away. Please regard this as a symptom, not as a disease, and a symptom of an underlying problem that can be reversed in many cases. First of all, avoid alcohol, which is a great irritant to the bladder sphincter. Avoid caffeine, which causes increased urination. Caffeine is not just in coffee, it's also found in cola beverages, chocolate, and many over-the-counter medications. Make sure you're not taking caffeine in any form. Smoking also causes irritation of the bladder, and "smoker's cough" can cause bladder leaking when the whole body goes into reflex spasm from the cough.

Maintain an optimum diet, which will help you lose excess weight, this itself will help take the pressure off the abdomen and the bladder to reduce incontinence. Your diet should also help you have normal bowel movements; the pressure from constipation can irritate the bladder. The proper diet would be high in fiber, with enough fluid to keep the fiber from making you more constipated. It would include a lot of vegetables, moderate amounts of fruit, whole grains, nuts, seeds, legumes, fish and chicken. Keep a food diary of what you eat and drink, the times that you urinate, and the times you have incontinence. After a week or so, you may see a pattern: a relationship between what you eat and how often your bladder leaks. It may be a simple matter of drinking too much fluid. However, dehydrating yourself is not the answer to this condition.

The advice that urologists give for this condition includes what is called "double voiding:" after you urinate, remain on the toilet and wait for any excess urine that remains to leave the bladder. You can apply gentle pressure over the pubic bone, run the water tap, or bend forward a bit to encourage all the urine to run out of the bladder. Some people hold back when they have to urinate. At a seminar, meeting, or social event, they ignore nature's call and hold their bladder until it becomes too full. If this is done too frequently it can weaken the sphincter muscles. Some people don't even know they have to go to the bathroom until they start to feel pain in the abdomen above the pubic bone.

Those at risk for incontinance should begin a "bladder drill," using the toilet at regular, structured intervals. This will help awareness of what it feels like to have smaller amounts in the bladder instead of the big, stretching pain that comes when the bladder is overfull. Retraining the bladder like this seems to set the bladder capacity to a better level for emptying. We urinate an average of every two and a half to five hours. In the bladder drill, if you try to void every hour, then over the next month or so, increase the time between voiding.

Exercises that are especially important for the bladder are called the Kegel exercises. Dr. Kegel felt that the bladder sphincter muscles, just like any other muscles, could be exercised and trained. The instructions are to pretend you're tightening the muscles around the anus, and then pretend you're holding back the urine, this identifies the two groups of muscles that you're going to be working on. Then starting at the anus, tighten those muscles, and then proceed forward, tightening the muscles at the urethra, hold this to a count of four, then release. Dr. Kegel advised this be done for two minutes, three times a day, or at least a hundred times daily. You can do the Kegel exercise when you're waiting at a traffic light, for a bus, or anywhere at all.

No one knows when you're doing "Kegels" and they are very helpful.

Infections

ᕙ Look at the chapters on **Colds and Flus, Bladder Infections, Bronchitis, Diarrhea, Earaches, Epstein-Barr, Kidney Disease, Prostate Problems, Pyorrhea, Sinus Infections and Vaginitis.**

The **First Aid** section includes treatment for skin and wound infections, and also for burns. However, the single most important treatment for wounds is proper cleaning of the wound and proper soaking. To clean a dirty wound, use dilute hydrogen peroxide. This substance will bubble on contact with pus. After all the dirt is removed *calendula, echineacea, hypericum* or *goldenseal* tincture diluted, about 10 drops per 4 oz. of water can be used to wash and pack a wound. If a wound is producing a lot of pus, like a boil, it is wise to try and keep it open to maximize draining. The best way to accomplish this is to obtain sterile gauze from the drugstore and dip it in the above herbal water and pack it into the wound. As the wound is cleaned of the debris, fresh live tissue is formed so that it will heal from the base up.

For soaking, use hot water with salt or Epsom salts. Soaking is done several times a day. For poultices, use moist bread, clay, or boiled herbs such as *comfrey.*

Of course if there are red streaks going away from a wound, suspect blood poisoning and seek medical advice and maybe an antibiotic. If you take an antibiotic, be sure and use *acidophilus* by mouth to replace the good bacteria.

Infertility—Female

ᕙ In the 1930s, Weston Price D.D.S. and Francis Pottenger M.D., did an interesting study on cats which may have implications for human infertility. The cats who were fed an optimum cat diet of raw meat and milk fared well, but the cats whose food was cooked and pasteurized could produce no live births by the third generation. I'm not suggesting that mothers eat raw meat and milk, but just consider how much "live" food you do eat. By making a substantial part of the diet raw fruits and vegetables, sprouts, whole grains, nuts and seeds, you are passing on the beneficial nutrients and enzymes of live foods to your child.

In modern society, there are many causes of infertility. Diet is one, environmental pollution is another. Drug intake is another, including the use of the birth control pill.

In my practice, I have counselled teens whose friends have gone to birth control clinics and been freely handed the pill. These girls may not have even started their periods, yet they are given a daily hormone that basically tricks the body into thinking it is pregnant. We may now be seeing the result of this practice. After ten years of artificial hormone intake, the body may not be able to jump start its own hormonal cascade. The daily levels of estrogen and progesterone have long since shut down the pituitary gland's production of FSH and LH, which prepare the follicles in the ovaries to become eggs.

Quite often, these women are then given huge doses of more hormones to jolt the pituitary into action. Often multiple births can result, with unknown repercussions on the health of the child.

Vitamin and mineral imbalances may also be created by the use of the pill. The B vitamins, including folic acid, are depleted, since they are used as coenzymes in the biochemical breakdown of the hormones in the pill. Most of this processing occurs in the liver. The liver is thus diverted from other work to perform this function.

Folic acid is crucial to prevent neural tube defects in the newborn. But it is even more crucial to create the neural tube in the first place. Many of the first trimester miscarriages may be occurring due to nonviability of the fetus from folic acid deficiency.

Folic acid can be found in all green vegetables.

When one reads of the nutrient needs for conception and pregnancy, almost every nutrient discovered is implicated. Therefore, the best advice is to maintain an excellent diet of whole foods, as close to their natural state as possible. Also make sure there are no underlying allergies, Candidiasis or mineral deficiencies by having blood tests and a hair mineral analysis. Avoid coffee, alcohol, and cigarettes for obvious reasons of toxicity. Don't do more than an hour of strenuous exercise a day because it can burn off too much fat which is necessary for proper hormone production and ovulation. Douching should be avoided, since it changes the normal vaginal pH.

Of course, the normal tests for infertility must be done to rule out any anatomical abnormalities. Make sure there is no underlying reason for the body not being able to sustain new life. If the body is chronically ill or chronically allergic, then it is probable that it will not direct its energies toward creating new life until it has a good lifeforce to sustain it.

Long use of the birth control pill is often to blame for conception difficulties. Give your body at least six months to rebalance before trying to conceive. A good vitamin and mineral supplement that emphasizes the B vitamins, especially folic acid, is essential during this period to prevent spina bifida.

Infertility—Male

এ It is very important to understand that males contribute 50% to fertility and that their diet and lifestyle can have an effect on their semen and sperm count. This means men should avoid smoking, decrease sugar, coffee, alcohol and refined foods in the diet. An excellent diet will achieve optimum results.

Men should also avoid tight underwear. The testicles are meant to hang away from the body and they make sperm best at a lower temperature than body temperature. Hot tubs should also be avoided.

If the sperm count is low and a possible cause of infertility, there are several supplements that can be used. A low sperm count can be increased with *zinc*, chelated or picolinate form, 50 mg daily for one month; then 25 mg daily. Agglutination of sperm can be balanced with *vitamin C*, 1000 mg per day, and sperm motility can be enhanced with *arginine*, an amino acid, 1 gram four times per day.

Insomnia

✇ These days, people are often so wound up before going to bed that it is difficult to settle the mind or the body into sleep. If this is the case, it is important to relax before bedtime. Avoid coffee or alcohol or a late dinner. Don't do strenuous exercise at this time (although intercourse often helps one sleep). Take a hot bath with Epsom salts, play some quiet music. Perform this type of ritual before bed so that the mind begins to slow down and turn off as a prelude to sleep. Some people play a relaxation tape while lying in bed. Daily exercise is also very important to achieve good sleep.

Sleep specialists recommend that people get up and change beds if sleep has not come within one-half hour or get up and leave the bedroom and read etc. until fatigue or tiredness sets in. Then return to the bedroom to sleep. Don't use your bedroom for anything else but sleep. Set your alarm and get up at the same time each morning. Don't nap during the day. Go to bed at a reasonable hour the next night. These instructions, followed to the letter, should reprogram your body to sleep properly.

A supplement that can help insomnia due to anxiety and hyper states is *tryptophan*, an amino acid, 500 mg 1 to 2 at bedtime with vegetable juice. This should not be taken within three hours of taking protein. The tryptophan scare a few years ago was with a specific batch of tryptophan that caused an allergic reaction and fever. The problem was with the binders and fillers in a new process using genetic engineering at a company in Japan, not with the tryptophan itself. Tryptophan should be available in the U.S. by prescription soon.

Herbal remedies include tinctures of *skullcap*, 10 to 15 drops in a few ounces of water, or capsules combining *hops, valerian* and *skullcap*, 1 to 2 at bedtime. One of the many homeopathic treatments is *Coffea* 6c, 4 drops, one to two doses at 15 minute intervals before bedtime to quiet an overactive mind.

Kidney Disease

~ This condition is usually diagnosed when a blood test shows a protein spill in the urine. By the time the kidneys are symptomatic with pain, kidney disease may be well advanced. Kidney infections may result from untreated bladder infections, by back flow of the urine up into the kidneys, by taking toxic medications or drugs, or by precipitation of minerals as kidney stones. Strengthening treatment of the kidneys include *nettle, parsley, uva ursi,* and *juniper berries*. These teas can be taken periodically to help keep the kidneys strong.

Excess animal protein puts a strain on the kidneys, so foods of this nature should be severely limited.

Kidney Stones

~ This condition, once it has occurred, has a high probability of recurring. The actual kidney stone attack is best treated in the hospital, but often it is only treated with pain-killers, rest, and time. There are new methods of removing kidney stones surgically that are less invasive than earlier ones. A small instrument can be inserted up the urethra into the kidney area, and the stone visualized on x-ray. An instrument can then crush the stone and the debris can be urinated out. There are also ultrasound machines that can be directed at the area of the stone; in this case, sonic waves crush the stone.

However, prevention is obviously the best treatment. Some people get kidney stones through dehydration in times of stress, or from not drinking enough water. A kidney or bladder infection can be a warning signal. Drink plenty of fluids to prevent the buildup of the minerals that can cause the kidney stones.

Over 40 percent of all kidney stones are made up of calcium or calcium combinations. The way to prevent this from occurring is not necessarily by limiting your calcium foods, but by taking in enough magnesium to balance with the calcium. We seem to eat more calcium-rich foods than magnesium-rich foods. Calcium occurs in dairy products, green, leafy vegetables, nuts, seeds, and fish. Magnesium occurs in whole grains, as well as in the green, leafy vegetables.

Over 50 percent of all stones are calcium oxalate stones; oxalates are found in foods such as rhubarb, raw spinach, parsley, chocolate and tea. These foods should be limited. A high intake of protein can also increase calcium and phosphorus in the urine, which may lead to calcium stones. Salt can also cause precipitation of calcium in the kidneys. A rare, possible source of overproduction of oxalates is thought to be from high doses of vitamin C. This has been researched by many people, but even with extremely high intakes of up to 100 grams of vitamin C per day in AIDS patients there has been no incidence of kidney stones.

The treatments for kidney stone prevention include *magnesium* (300 to 400 mg daily) and *vitamin B6*. B6 can lower the amount of oxalate in the urine and it is a natural diuretic, which increases the flushing of the kidneys. Dosages of 50 mg per day are often recommended. *Vitamin A* and *beta carotene* are very helpful for mucous membrane production and healing, so they help maintain the urinary tract lining. Simply eating a carrot or two a day will provide you with enough vitamin A.

Lactose Intolerance

๛ Some people believe that cow's milk is only for baby calves and that humans should not consume dairy products; they say we are the only mammals who take milk past the age of weaning. For some people, this may be good advice, especially for those millions of adults who do not have the necessary lactase enzymes to digest the milk. Africans are especially apt to be lactose-intolerant and over 80 percent of them cannot digest milk. I have always been struck by the terrible irony of sending dry, powdered milk to people suffering from famine, or after catastrophes in Africa, when this product will actually make these people sicker. As many as 30 percent of whites are also lactose-intolerant. The diagnosis is through blood tests or by a breath test. The blood test will often confirm symptoms in the gastrointestinal tract, such as diarrhea, cramps, gas, or even constipation.

It's amazing, though, how many people are not aware of their lactose intolerance. Some people are thrown off by the fact that when they eat dairy with other foods, they don't have as many symptoms or don't have any symptoms at all. This can be because the digestion time is increased, so that if they have some enzymes available to digest the milk, they are not used up all at once. Eating yogurt can be a way to take dairy products without getting any symptoms; yogurt has much less lactose content than milk. If you make your own yogurt, instead of incubating it for only 12 hours, continue the incubation for 24 hours and more of the lactose will be broken down. If you decide to avoid dairy products, take a *calcium/magnesium* supplement. Taking excess calcium without magnesium might be a cause of future kidney stones. Avoid supplements like Tums, which have antacid properties which greatly decrease the absorption of the calcium. Foods rich in calcium are listed in the chapter on **Osteoporosis**. The calcium-magnesium ratio in supplements is usually 2-to-1, and the total daily intake of calcium should be around 1,000 mg, so check the sources that you take every day, and make up the balance with supplements.

There is a product on the market now called Lactaid, available in tablets or drops, to put in your milk. Lactase-treated cheeses are also available with up to 90 percent of the lactose digested. However, for people who are extremely allergic to milk, the 10 percent that is left over could still be a problem.

One of the conditions that a person can develop with lactose intolerance or the over-consumption of dairy products is Candidiasis. Lactose is a disaccharide made up of glucose and galactose. When this breaks down, you then have glucose sugar available, which can have the same effect on yeast organisms as refined sugar. The discussion on Candidiasis in this book might by useful. You may find that avoiding dairy eases your symptoms, especially if you also avoid sugar, bread with yeast, and fermented foods.

Leg Cramps

⮂ A condition commonly called "charlie horse" can cause excruciating pain usually in the calf of the leg or the foot and is associated with a *calcium* or *magnesium* deficiency. *Vitamin E* can help prevent a condition called restless legs. This occurs in bed at night when the legs twitch and jump almost uncontrollably causing insomnia and fatigue. Poor circulation can aggravate both of these conditions. Poor circulation in the calf muscles leading to chronic pain is called intermittent claudication. (If blood vessels in the heart are blocked, the pain is called angina; blocked vessels to the penis lead to impotence.) An acutely inflamed, swollen and painful calf can be caused by a blood clot which needs emergency care.

For chronic intermittent claudication, first stop smoking. Next start walking. Alternating warm and cold foot baths several times can help. For poor circulation which results in cold feet, don't use hot water, heating pads or hot water bottles, as you could burn your feet. Choose proper foot gear and take good care of your feet. When the circulation is poor, cuts and infections don't heal.

In children, leg cramps or pains are sometimes related to growing pains. *Vitamin E* supplementation, 400 to 800 I.U. will often alleviate this problem as well.

Liver Disease

࿔ The most common liver condition is hepatitis. There is infectious hepatitis A and serum hepatitis B; the treatment for both is similar. High doses of *vitamin C*, up to 10 grams a day has an antiviral effect. Protein in the diet is important; it is difficult for strict vegetarians to overcome hepatitis. Herbal tinctures of *black Russian radish*, 10 drops in water twice a day, and homeopathic *Cheladonia* 6c 4 drops three times a day, are also indicated. Castor oil packs can be placed over the liver to enhance the lymphatic clearing of toxins. The liver can also respond to other viral infections by releasing liver enzymes into the blood. The treatment is the same. For mononucleosis, add the homeopathic remedy *Cistus canidenses* 6c, 4 drops three times a day.

Menopausal Symptoms

࿔ Menopause is a natural occurrence. The female hormones decline after the age of 45 and periods cease between 45 and 55. One thing that the periods do is flush toxins from the body. I often wonder if the cessation of regular bleeding is one reason why more women develop arthritic-type symptoms during the menopause. Perhaps they are holding onto more toxins, which then can deposit in the joint spaces. I, therefore, think it is important for women in the menopausal years to start some form of detoxification. (See the chapter on **Detoxification**.)

In Japan and in third world countries, women do not seem to experience the same symptoms of menopause that women do in North America. There is very little hot flushing, depression or mood change in this normal phase of a woman's life. All these symptoms can be looked upon as either dietary, psychological, or psychosocial.

First and foremost, women should strive to maintain an excellent diet. As a person ages, it is important to cut back on protein intake, especially not having protein at the evening meal. One should also increase enzymes in the body with the use of such foods as papaya or pineapple or to take *enzyme tablets* to aid digestion and food breakdown. Exercise is also important to keep the bones strong and the heart circulatory system healthy.

I am not an advocate of hormonal replacement therapy. Estrogen stimulates growth including that of cancer. If a woman is diagnosed with cancer, she is immediately taken off estrogen.

Cancer starts as one cell and, if there are hormones stimulating it or a weakened immune system, it will flourish. I would not want to prescribe hormones to someone who may have the beginning of cancer and possibly hasten it. There are many natural remedies to try before resorting to synthetic hormones.

One such treatment is high doses of *folic acid*. This B vitamin is getting a lot of attention in medical research. It has been shown to help heal cervical dysplasia, and it alleviates the symptoms of menopause. The book to read on this topic is Dr. Robert Atkins' *The Health Revolution*. The dosage may be from 10 mg to 80 mg per day. This must be obtained by prescription and under a doctor's supervision.

For vaginal dryness, try *K-Y Jelly* as a lubricant and *vitamin E oil* for vaginal healing. Some formulas that are available contain *evening primrose oil, vitamin A* and *vitamin E*. For specific symptoms, such as flooding that can periodically occur with blood clots and heavy bleeding, the *bioflavinoids* are especially important, 1000 mg. 1 to 2 per day during the flooding or before an expected period. This supplement heals the capillaries lining the uterus. If this symptom comes after having missed a period for many months, please see your doctor.

Hot flushes which are related to hormonal shifts can be treated by making sure the adrenal glands are supported in their production of female hormones as they take over from the ovaries. Hot flushes occur less in women who have regular intercourse (at least once weekly).

If the adrenal glands are exhausted, it might be more difficult for this hormone production to occur and support must be given in the form of *desiccated adrenal*, 1 to 2 tablets twice a day, mid-morning and mid-afternoon; *pantothenic acid*, a B vitamin that supports the adrenal glands, 500 mg three times a day; *vitamin C*, which supports the adrenal glands, 1000 mg two times a day; *vitamin E*, 400 I.U., 1 to 2 per day will aid the circulation and the liver. Ginseng as well as black cohosh can be useful herbs. *Red Korean ginseng* is the best form, 2 to 4 capsules a day; *black cohosh* in tincture form, 10 drops, two to three doses in water per day.

Homeopathic remedies such as *Sepia* and *Pulsatilla* are very important for menopause. Consult a homeopathic text or a homeopathic doctor for remedies targeted to your own symptoms. Calcium and magnesium are very important even before menopause to prevent osteoporosis. They can be introduced and used at any time after age 30 and should be continued indefinitely; *calcium* 1000 mg and *magnesium* 500 to 1000 mg per day (if no dairy products are eaten) are the recommended requirements.

Exercise is also very important. Yoga, tai chi, swimming and walking are the best forms of exercise. Apart from diet and nutrition, attitude plays a great role in any of life's transitions.

Some women look forward to menopause as a time when the children have left home and they are now free to pursue careers and goals that were impossible before because of responsibilities at home. Therefore, they embrace this time in their life with renewed vigor, interest and excitement. It can be a more carefree time when women can do what they want to do, not what family or society dictates.

The time of menopause also corresponds with Jung's mid-life stage. The previous years have been outward: seeking, accomplishing, doing. The focus now seems to be more inward: toward being and creativity.

Menstrual Pain

 The medical term for this condition is dysmenorrhea. Painful periods are caused by irregular contractions felt to be initiated by prostaglandins. This has led to treatment with anti-prostaglandin drugs such as Ponstel. The natural treatment would be *evening primrose oil* which enhances the type of prostaglandins that inhibit these contractions; treatment is 4 to 6 per day throughout the month to prepare for the menstrual period.

Another treatment is with calcium and magnesium which help stabilize the contractions of the uterus. Dosage is 300 mg of calcium and 150 mg of magnesium every one to two hours during the day when the contractions occur. These pills can be taken as you would pain medication during the painful days. Some women may be deficient in calcium and magnesium and need this supplement on a regular basis, especially if avoiding dairy. Recommended daily dosage for young adults is 1000 to 1200 mg calcium and 500 to 600 mg magnesium. Check with your doctor for dosages according to your individual needs. Make sure there is no *vitamin D* in these tablets to avoid excess intake of D. Cutting out coffee, alcohol, meat, sugar, dairy, salt and white bread 7 to 10 days before the period can be very helpful in reducing menstrual cramps.

Castor oil packs and hot water bottles on the abdomen can be very soothing. Use several tablespoons of castor oil on an old hand towel. Soak oil into the towel and cover the lower abdomen with the towel and cover with plastic. Heat with a hot water bottle. Leave the pack on for at least one hour at a time. Hot baths with Epsom salts are also very helpful. Exercise is also very important to help stabilize contractions so swim, walk or stretch during the pain. Intercourse can help as well.

There are several homeopathic remedies that are useful for painful periods. Use *Mag. phos.* for the type of pain that is better curled up in a ball with a hot water bottle pressing against the right side. The dosage is four drops 6c or 30c every half hour. *Colocynthis* is for more intense sharp stabbing pain better with pressure than with heat and more on the left side; the mood is bitter and irritable. *Cimicifuga* is for severe cramps across the abdomen, down the legs, and for back aches; the patient is hysterical, irritable, and achy. This is taken, 6c or 30c, 4 drops every hour while in pain. There are many remedies for this condition. A homeopathic book or better still, a homeopathic doctor should be consulted if the first few remedies do not achieve the desired result.

Mononucleosis

(SEE EPSTEIN-BARR)

Multiple Sclerosis

This degeneration of the myelin sheath surrounding the nerves can occur in any nerve of the body, leading to widespread, non-specific, and confusing symptoms. The cause of MS is unknown and, at this point, the treatment or cure is unknown. There is a consensus that there is no one treatment for MS but a variety of treatments that can help alleviate some of the symptoms.

Often, the diagnosis can take several years to confirm. In that time, a patient can experience eye, bladder and muscle symptoms. If the bladder is affected and a person begins to get bladder infections, antibiotic overuse can lead to an overgrowth of yeast in the system. The toxins from the yeast will irritate the nerves of the body even more, thus increasing the symptoms of MS.

Anxiety about what is causing the symptoms and not having a diagnosis can also cause or mimic MS symptoms. For example, hyperventilation can cause tingling and numbness in the extremities, just as MS does. Some research has shown that allergenic foods can cause antigen-antibody reactions in the system which can further irritate the nerves, muscles and joints.

The natural treatment for MS entails dietary manipulation to avoid the major allergenic foods: dairy, wheat and perhaps all the gluten grains which include wheat, rye, oats and barley. Sugar and alcohol are excluded also. Roy Swank, M.D., has been treating MS patients for over 40 years and has found that avoiding wheat and dairy can stabilize a person and prevent progression of the disease. His book is called *The Multiple Sclerosis Cookbook*.

People who have been treated with cortisone for their flare-ups and antibiotics for the bladder symptoms are advised to go on Candida treatment. (See the chapter on **Candidiasis**.) With a hypo-allergenic diet and a Candida diet, a great many of the MS symptoms can be relieved or alleviated. Homeopathy seems to have a place in the treatment of MS but the remedies would be constitutional remedies which can only be given after a complete history has been taken by a homeopathic doctor.

Nails

&. Nails and their abnormalities are related to many different deficiencies. Brittle nails indicate an iron deficiency and decreased circulation. Brittle, ridged, thin nails indicate Raynaud's syndrome in which there is decreased circulation during cold weather or during periods of stress. Spoon shaped nails with a concavity indicate an *iron* deficiency. Brittle nails can also indicate overuse of solvents and detergents. White spots on the nails indicate *zinc* deficiency or, more rarely, a loss of protein in the urine. In teenage diets, zinc is very low and it is required to metabolize the junk food diets so many young people eat. Yellowish nails indicate lymphatic congestion, respiratory congestion or deficiency in *vitamin E*. Yellow toenails, red patches and bruising around the nails indicate diabetes. Dark nails can indicate a *B12* deficiency. A white cuticle with a dark tip is an indication of chronic kidney disease. Whitish nails indicate liver or kidney disease or anemia. Horizontal ridges on the nails indicate protein or zinc deficiency. Vertical lines on the nails indicate *iron, calcium* or *magnesium* deficiency.

Nausea

꿈 In my practice, I see many people with nausea, often because of Candidiasis. (See the chapter on **Candidiasis**.) Or it could be from the toxicity that can occur when the body is completely overloaded with junk food. Imagine a barrel filled to the top with oil, dirt and debris; anything else that goes in assumes the character of the debris. Sometimes people are so toxic that any food that they take in just adds to their toxicity. In this case, people have to detoxify and cleanse before they do anything else. Good food and excellent supplements are useless in the face of a toxic overload. Read the chapter on **Detoxification** to help with this. If the nausea is due to pregnancy, read the chapter on **Pregnancy**.

The best remedy for nausea while exploring the above chapters or if the nausea is caused by motion sickness is *ginger tea* or *ginger capsules*. Acupuncture is also very helpful because it can work on the vagus nerve, which may be irritated by stomach acidity and give a constant nausea reflex. However, in most cases, nausea is only a symptom of a bigger problem.

Neck Pain

∂∿ The problem of neck pain is extremely common among North Americans. It has to do with the way we sit at our desk with our neck bent forward or shoulders slumped and our brows scrunched up in concentration. It starts in the shoulders and moves up into the neck. It can feel like we have just been in a motor vehicle accident and suffered whiplash. Muscle spasms in the neck can be very severe. The best treatments are heat or ice, and if both give some relief, they can be used alternately. Massage is very helpful and you can do a reasonable self-massage that can relieve the neck. Lying on two tennis balls tied up in a sock and positioned at the base of the skull can relieve pressure. However, do so carefully so that you don't cause more pain. To avoid neck pain, make sure you sit with good back support. I personally find that the kneeling chair is helpful. It has two levels of cushioning: one you kneel on, and the other you rest your buttocks on. By kneeling forward on your knees, you redistribute your weight, which produces a new forward center of gravity. This maintains your body in an upright posture. When you're working at a computer, as so many people do today, make sure your computer is at eye level and that you neither have to look up nor down. An accessory is available which elevates the computer screen—or you can stack up several telephone books.

When you lift any heavy object, be sure that you're bending at the knees and not putting a strain on your back and neck. Sleeping for six to eight hours in the wrong position can aggravate neck problems. Choose a firm mattress. Use a rolled-up towel under your neck, or find a neck pillow or cervical pillow which puts proper support under your neck. Never sleep on your stomach; the best position is either on your back, or curled up in the fetal position. If your neck is very stiff or you feel tenderness in certain areas, you might want to check with a qualified chiropractor for treatment. You might be advised to get x-rays to diagnose any problems with your vertebrae. If your neck pain comes from a motor vehicle accident, be sure you are under the care of a medical doctor.

Night Blindness

ﾨ This condition is due to a vitamin A deficiency, so the treatment is very simple: take *vitamin A* or *beta carotene*. The best form is that found in food, and the sources are yellow vegetables such as carrots, yams and squash, or green, leafy vegetables, such as kale, spinach, and broccoli. High doses of vitamin A can cause side-effects. Never take more than 40,000 I.U. per day. The usual dosage is 10,000 I.U. Beta carotene, which is the precursor for vitamin A, does not produce side effects, and it is the beta carotene source that is found in vegetables.

Nosebleed

ﾨ Nosebleeds occur more often in the dry winter months due to the drying of the nasal membranes which leaves them susceptible to cracking and bleeding. To avoid this, humidify your living space, especially your bedroom, so that you have more moisture in the air to protect against the dryness.

Nosebleeds are often connected with more than dryness alone; a winter cold can bring on a lot of nasal mucous and irritation, with the consequent nose-blowing that sets the stage for the dryness, then the cracking and bleeding. Also, inhaled allergies to dust and mites, and even food allergies, such as to dairy and wheat, can cause extra mucous in the nose. Therefore, the vicious cycle is set up that results in breakage or tears in the membranes inside the nose, which can take up to a week to heal. Usually, people can't leave their nose alone for more than an hour without blowing out the mucous or even picking at the crusts, and it will require much longer periods in order to heal a damaged area in the nose. The more you stick your fingers into the nose and pick at it, the more you are susceptible to nasal boils. These are usually staphylococcal bacterial infections which start with a very painful swelling in the nose, form pus, and then dry and crust.

The nose is very sensitive, and the treatment for this vicious cycle is to leave the nose alone except for using *vitamin E oil*, several times a day, to help lubricate the nose lining and heal the scabs. If you do get a staphylococcal boil, you will need an antibiotic ointment, used several times a day, to kill that bacteria.

The vitamin and mineral treatments for nosebleed include *vitamin C with bioflavinoids, zinc, calcium* and *magnesium*. Drugs that interfere with clotting by thinning the blood include aspirin, as well as drugs that are taken specifically to thin the blood. Sometimes the side effect of these medications is nosebleeds, but you can overcome that if you will follow the advised recommendations. Not everybody taking these medications has nosebleeds.

Obesity

This is a condition of civilization and there seems to be no easy answer or quick fix. You have to explore the emotional and physical reasons for being overweight and work on both areas. On the physical nutritional side, food allergies often play a part. You may be eating foods to which the body is allergic; this can lead to excess fluid retention, your body's way of diluting the antigen-antibody toxins. Therefore, food allergy testing may be helpful for those who have "tried every diet in the book."

Small frequent meals are important for weight loss rather than starving through the day and making up for it with one large meal at night. If you only eat one large meal a day, you may actually gain weight because the body is designed to metabolize, digest, and break down what it needs in the few hours following the meal. Therefore, if one large meal is consumed, only a portion of the food will be metabolized and utilized and the excess will go into fat storage.

Also make sure you get enough exercise. Most people are unable to lose weight—and keep it off—unless they are on a good exercise program of vigorous walking, swimming or bicycling.

What about fasting to achieve weight loss? This is not the best way. It is important to change lifestyle and habits to achieve lasting success. Some people, however, whose allergies to foods contribute to their weight problems, might try a fast which includes *hypoallergenic protein powder* with *psyllium seed* or another bulking agent plus vegetables for a period of three to ten days. This will get rid of fluid weight and clear the body of possible allergenic foods. Then one can begin challenge testing the possible allergenic foods. (See the chapter on **Allergies**.) *UltraBalance protein powder* or *blue-green algae protein powder* or *UltraClear protein powder* are available through your naturopath or health food distributor.

When people go on fasts or diets they often feel so sick within two to three days that they quit the program, and all their good intentions fly out the window. Like caffeine or cigarette withdrawal, when you stop eating foods you are addicted to, the body starts flushing the poisons or toxins from those foods out of your system. As these toxins are released, especially from fat cells where they are stored, you can feel really bad with headaches, cramps, diarrhea, or fatigue. So any diet must be started slowly; you must drink lots of water to flush out poisons and above all, avoid constipation. You are actually detoxifying your body.

Osteoporosis

 Osteoporosis is more and more in the news, probably because our population is aging. Also there is a big push from pharmaceutical companies to use estrogen replacement therapy to help strengthen the bones. Others are stressing calcium supplementation for the bones. All this information is quite varied and complex and is often not completely researched and leaves the public not really knowing how to proceed.

Osteoporosis means a thinning of the bones. If a bone is not exercised, it will automatically begin being reabsorbed. Space astronauts discovered this when they were in weightless flight. The most important advice is to maintain an optimum level of exercise to avoid reabsorption of the bone. Avoid alcohol which interferes with bone formation. Smoking lowers estrogen which adds to osteoporosis risk. Coffee also affects the bones adversely; it hastens calcium excretion probably by acting like a diuretic.

In countries with lower protein intake, osteoporosis is not a problem. Protein, especially meat with its high phosphorus content, causes calcium loss. Phosphates in soft drinks also seem to be a problem as they bind calcium and take it out of the body.

In terms of calcium replacement therapy for osteoporosis, it must be acknowledged that bones are made up of a multitude of minerals and nutrients and treatment should include all of them. These would be *calcium, magnesium, zinc, copper, mucopolysaccharides, chondroitin sulphates* and many of the *B vitamins* that are important for the enzymatic production of the bone. Most of the studies of osteoporosis will take one nutrient or modality and try to see if it prevents bone loss. In the individual case, it is important to assess and maintain all modalities. With regard to estrogen replacement, again there is no one thing that will help bone loss. When someone has true and obvious estrogen deficiencies and can only be helped with estrogen supplementation, then the hormone should be used. However, menopause is a natural transition in one's life and need not be medicated. (See the chapter on **Menopause**.)

Since many people avoid dairy for reasons of lactose intolerance, allergies, diarrhea, constipation or because of its fat content, here is a list of non-dairy sources of calcium taken from Joy Underwood's excellent book *Nourishing Your Body*.

FOOD	MG. CALCIUM
Vegetables	
1 cup cooked dried beans (white, kidney, soy, etc.)	95–110
½ cup cooked beet greens	157
1 medium stalk broccoli	158
½ cup cooked spinach	88
1 cup cooked turnip greens	126
½ cup cooked kale	103
½ cup cooked collards	110
½ cup cooked dandelion greens	147
1 cup bok choy cabbage	252
Baked Goods	
1 medium corn muffin	96
1 slice whole wheat bread	50
1 medium waffle	76
½ cup soy flour	132
1 tbsp. blackstrap molasses	140
Seafood	
20 medium oysters	300
6 scallops	115
7 sardines with bones	393
¾ can clams	62
½ can salmon with bones	284
Nuts and Seeds	
½ cup almonds	175
½ cup brazil nuts	128
½ cup sesame seeds	76
Fruit	
½ cup rhubarb, cooked	200

Phlebitis

෯ This occurs when a blood-clot forms in a deep vein of the legs. The reasons for it include intake of the birth control pill or long periods of immobility, such as during air travel or bedrest following surgical procedures or accidents. The best treatment is prevention, of course, and optimal diet, which keeps the blood from becoming too thick with cholesterol and triglycerides, as well as getting plenty of exercise. If you have a family history of phlebitis or have had an occurrence already, you must not smoke. Read the chapters on **Cholesterol** and **Atherosclerosis,** to get more information on how to take care of your veins and arteries.

Poison Ivy

ᔑ The best thing to do is to avoid poison ivy and to know what it looks like. Once you have contacted poison ivy, every effort should be made to isolate that area of the skin and not touch, rub or press it up against any other area of the skin or clothing which can retain the resin and pass the allergic reaction along. I have even had cases of patients who blistered after handling an old, dried, pressed specimen of poison ivy.

The treatment, if it can be accomplished on the spot, is to locate a *jewel weed* plant and rub the plant over the affected area. If you live in a poison ivy region, make sure you learn how to identify both plants. At home, wash the area with warm, soapy water and never touch the blisters without washing your hands. Also, take *Rhus tox.*, a homeopathic remedy for poison ivy by mouth, either 30c or 200c hourly. Keep the area dry and apply *calamine lotion.*

Pregnancy

ᔑ There are many good books available on nutritional and herbal advice for pregnancy; a particular favorite is by Susun Weed, called *The Child Bearing Years*. Before conception, the most important thing is to make sure, by blood test, that you are protected against rubella (German measles). If acquired during pregnancy, Rubella can harm the fetus. The immunity conferred by natural infection during childhood is the best; second best is immunization against the disease. One should not get pregnant in the three to six months following immunization for rubella.

Immunizations themselves are controversial and the recommendation is to take homeopathic remedies such as *Thuja* 6c after the shot to prevent side effects. *Vitamin C*, the *B vitamins* and *zinc* are also important to help the body deal with the foreign material injected.

That having been accomplished, a thorough physical exam and blood tests to determine the status of the hemoglobin, thyroid, blood sugar, iron and the liver should also be done before conception. The diet of both parents should be optimum and avoidance of coffee, alcohol and cigarette smoke is best because all these factors have been shown to produce adverse effects on the growth and health of the fetus. Nutritional advice during pregnancy is to maintain a high fiber diet to avoid constipation, and to eat plenty of vegetables, fish, chicken, nuts, whole grains and seeds. One must avoid eating too much fruit because there are cases of women getting gestational diabetes just from the overconsumption of fruit.

Once pregnant, the best position to take when sleeping is to lie on the left side so that the growing uterus is supported over the sigmoid colon. Lying on the back or right side can produce undue pressure on the great veins of the trunk of the body leading to the legs which can in turn cause varicose veins of the legs and varicosities of the labia as well as hemorrhoids. Another anatomical risk is hiatus hernia which is caused by the pressure of the enlarging uterus as it pushes the stomach up between the diaphragm.

The treatment for hiatus hernia or stomach pressure against the diaphragm is to eat small frequent meals; don't drink water with a meal because that bloats the stomach; don't lie down immediately after a meal; and have the area of the stomach massaged down and to the right in order to maintain the stomach in its proper position. See the chapter on **Digestion** for a discussion of hiatus hernia.

The supplements that are necessary during pregnancy are *iron,* for building up the blood (the best is chelated iron which is better absorbed than the ferrous irons), 25 to 50 mg per day; *folic acid,* 5 mg per day which prevents certain birth defects (this amount is now available only on prescription); a good *multiple vitamin* and *mineral* that has *vitamins A* and *D* and the *B vitamins* and *minerals. Calcium* and *magnesium* are required in addition, especially for non-dairy-eating mothers. The *calcium* requirement is 1200 to 1500 mg and half as much *magnesium.* Calcium and magnesium are best taken away from fiber in the evening.

For morning sickness try to eat and drink frequently to keep your blood sugar up. Some people feel morning sickness is a good sign of healthy hormone activity and a way for your body to turn against junk food at a time when you need the best for your baby. Avoid coffee, cigarettes, alcohol, sugar and fried foods. Snack on nuts and seeds and drink plenty of fluids. For morning sickness, *ginger* and *red raspberry leaf teas* are helpful; *vitamin B6* is also helpful, 100 to 300 mg per day.

The homeopathic remedies for morning sickness are:

Anacardium is for a pregnant woman who eats small amounts and gets a sinking feeling in the pit of her stomach, gas and bloating.

Cocculus is for being worse with motion, being unable to stand the sight or smell of food, or dizziness or sleep loss.

Colchicum is for being worse with the smell of meat, eggs or fried food and feeling cold from the inside out.

Pulsatilla is for upset stomach, gastric irritation; for when heavy foods aggravate the condition, for feeling helpless, moody, crying a lot and wanting something to eat but don't know what.

Sepia is for mental and emotional depression, irritability, persistent nausea and vomiting, yelling and hitting; worse with meat and eggs.

Ipecac is for constant nausea, complete disgust for even the thought of food; thirstlessness.

Ignatia is for cramps and spasms, knotted up stomach, hysterical behavior, sensitivity, edginess and irritability.

Nux vomica is for morning cramps and spasms, rashes, a toxic hang over, headache, nausea, irritability, feeling better in the afternoon.

All these remedies are given in a 6c potency, 4 drops every fifteen minutes to four hours. If one remedy doesn't work within two days, another remedy should be sought. If several fail to have effect, a homeopathic doctor should be consulted.

During pregnancy, a blood test should be taken for thyroid function. Sometimes, pregnancy can put an unnecessary strain on the thyroid which can result in deficiency. A repeat test should be done at the postnatal six-week checkup.

To prepare for labor, some women use *Caulophyllum,* 6 or 30c, several doses a day the last week or two before delivery. This can also be used during labor to help balance the contractions. *Arnica* is used during labor and after delivery for bruising or shock, 6 or 30c, one dose every half hour. *Aconite* can be used after a difficult labor, 200c, one to two doses. *Causticum* can also be used for urinary retention in the same dosage. *Rhus tox.* in 6 or 30c dosage can be used for the strain of pregnancy leading to stiffness, muscle aches and chilliness. *Staphasagria,* 6c or 30c, can be used for pain of the urethra especially if the patient has been catheterized. It is very important on the day of delivery or the day after to begin using 50 mg of *zinc* per day to replace the stores that are greatly diminished by delivery. This dosage should be taken for one month and then reduced to 25 mg per day for one more month. Zinc helps with wound healing, plus it is excellent in preventing postpartum depression. Zinc continues to be taken during breastfeeding in the *multiple vitamin* and *mineral.*

Premenstrual Syndrome

ৈ PMS is a hormonal condition of inappropriate fluid retention before the period that causes bloating, swelling, and weight
gain as well as psychological distress such as poor concentration, depression, irritability, anxiety and anger. Some women
can become so irritated that they become suicidal or homicidal.
Of course, these cases are as rare as they are extreme.

First of all, it would be helpful to keep a record of your
cycle and symptoms to determine whether it is in fact PMS. The
symptoms must occur from ovulation to the period and disappear at the onset of menses. The mere identification of one's
symptoms as being cyclical can help to alleviate some of the
discomfort. With simple rest and awareness, one knows that the
symptoms will subside in a few days and there's no need to get
too caught up in them.

Dietary advice includes avoiding foods which retain salt and
sugar and in turn will retain fluid. Avoid chips, sugar, desserts,
alcohol, tea, coffee, soft drinks and try to eat an optimum diet
of whole grains, nuts, seeds, vegetables, legumes, fish and
chicken.

The next step is to use *vitamin B6* to decrease fluid buildup,
100 mg one to three times a day from mid-cycle to the period.
Another supplement that is deficient in premenstrual syndrome
is *magnesium;* 300 mg a day is a good amount to continue all
month and can be taken with a *calcium* supplement of equal
strength. This is especially important for those women who suffer painful periods. *Evening primrose oil* is used for many of
the premenstrual symptoms, especially breast tenderness and can
also be used for painful periods. This is taken four to six capsules per day. A good all-round *vitamin* and *mineral* is also an
asset, especially for its B vitamin content to help balance the
use of extra *B6*.

I also use homeopathic remedies with my patients. The three simplest ones are:

Sepia which is for dark haired women who are angry and irritable and push people away; who feel better when they are dancing, feel their uterus is falling and heavy and suffer leg pains prior and during the period. This can be taken 6c, 4 drops three times a day 7 to 10 days before the period.

Pulsatilla is for blonde women who are weepy and inconsolable but who also may be changeable; that is they may appear angry and irritable one moment like a Sepia, and the next minute be in a flood of tears. The same dosage, 6c, 4 drops three times a day is used, 7 to 10 days before the period.

Natrum mur. is a good remedy for people who are salt cravers. These people retain a lot of fluid and they are "shut down," i.e., not wanting to get involved with anyone and quite often have suffered a heartache or major grief which keeps them behind a protective barrier. They are often good listeners and try to help others but never get involved. Again this remedy is 6c, 4 drops 3 times a day for 7 to 10 days before the period.

Usually the remedies are used for three to four cycles when a lot of symptoms abate. After that the remedies are only used as needed.

The most severe cases that don't entirely respond to the above suggested treatments may require a prescription of *progesterone* by rectal suspension. This is used in dosages of 200 mg, one dose every twelve hours, 10 days before the period. This has to be individualized for each patient and can vary up to a dose as high as 400 mg twice a day or starting as early as fourteen days before the period or starting as late as five days before the period. I have read in the literature that several clinics use progesterone on most patients, but my experience indicates that with charting, B6, diet, supplements and remedies, it is rare indeed that I have to use progesterone at all. In normal doses it does not seem to produce side effects but it is inconvenient and messy and patients would prefer not to use it if they have a choice.

Prostate Problems

ᗧ The prostate gland is located at the base of the penis and helps produce prostatic fluid that makes up part of the seminal fluid. The main mineral that helps the prostate function is zinc. For any prostate condition, *zinc* is important, 25–50 mg per day for one month and then reduced to 25 mg per day.

Prostate herbal formulas are available in most health food stores. They may include *saw palmetto berries, cornsilk, pumpkin seeds, uva ursi* and *buchu*. The homeopathic remedies used for the prostate are *Thuja, Coninum, Medorrhinum, Staphasagria,* and *Baryta carb*. Check the section in this book on **Remedies** for their description. All these remedies are fairly powerful constitutional remedies and would require a naturopath or homeopath for their administration. They are usually taken in the 6c potency for one month to see if the condition can be improved.

There are far too many men having prostate resection for benign enlargement. The side effects of this operation may include impotence, so this surgery should not be taken lightly. As well as the basic supplements mentioned, it is also important to have an optimum diet and avoid heavy fried, spicy, rich foods that can increase the toxic burden on the body.

Psoriasis

ᗧ Psoriasis occurs when the cells of the skin reproduce up to a hundred times faster than normal. When this occurs, the skin builds up in dry, flaky patches and causes a lot of irritation, itching, and embarrassment. Unfortunately, product advertisements for treating 'the heartbreak of psoriasis' make the public think of it as a horrible disease, and for some people it is. But for people with mild to moderate conditions, you can actually aggravate your psoriasis by fretting and worrying about the appearance of a new skin lesion.

Number one, try not to worry. Sun bathing helps a lot; even sun lamps are helpful but be careful because too much sun has side effects. Use sunscreen on the non-psoriasis areas to prevent sun damage in those exposed areas. Tar-soaps sold at drug stores seem to help slow down the production of psoriatic patches.

One supplement that helps this condition is zinc, which is depleted by the excessive cell production. *Zinc* is used in amounts of 25 to 50 mg. No more than 25 mg should be used on a long-term basis since excess zinc may lower copper levels. Supplements should also include high doses of *vitamin A* (up to 30,000 I.U. a day under a doctor's supervision); *vitamin E,* 400 I.U. one to two a day; *B complex,* 50 mg one to two a day; *trace minerals; alfalfa tablets; calcium, magnesium,* and *bioflavins* with *vitamin C. Lecithin* is also helpful as well as the essential fatty acids in *evening primrose oil* and *marine lipids.* These oils have anti-inflammatory properties and have a beneficial effect on normalizing body tissues including skin.

I have found in my practice that when people are treated for Candidiasis or allergies, their psoriasis begins to clear up. Check the chapters on these conditions in this book for more information. It seems that almost any skin condition can be aggravated by Candida overgrowth.

The diet that is important in the treatment of psoriasis includes lots of vegetables, moderate fruit, lots of nuts, whole grains, legumes, beans and peas, fish and chicken. The avoidance of saturated fats and refined foods such as pork, beef and baked goods will greatly help the outcome. You must pay attention to the acid balance of the body and avoid oranges which can give an over alkaline reaction. Use cranberry juice, prunes and plums, which are a bit more acidic. Avoid alcohol, smoking coffee and sugar.

Pyorrhea

ᔥ This gum inflammation results from inadequate dental hygiene. If plaque and food build up between the teeth, they can irritate the gums and lead to gum inflammation. Dental floss or tape are helpful as well as a water pik. A remedy that Edgar Cayce recommended was *Glycothymoline* which contains a solution of boric acid. In the acute stages rinse the mouth with a dilution of one part Glycothymoline to three parts water. In the chronic stage, or once the acute stage has passed, 2 to 3 drops of Glycothymoline in eight ounces of water shaken 50 times, can be used as a mouth rinse every night homeopathically to prevent plaque build up and pyorrhea. *Calcium* and *magnesium* are important for the proper maintenance of the gums as well as *bioflavins, vitamin* C and *zinc*. An optimum diet would also be beneficial.

Raynaud's Syndrome

ᔥ Raynaud's is the name given to a condition which causes blue or white discoloration of the fingers due to lack of sufficient oxygen or blood supply to the fingers. There is no known cause for this condition. The treatments are designed to keep the fingers warm and improve the circulation in the hands. Always wear gloves in cold weather; swinging the arms like a windmill to force blood into the fingertips is helpful. Have your doctor check your hemoglobin and iron to see if you have a deficiency of hemoglobin which can decrease your oxygenation. People with low thyroids can have a lower body temperature so read the chapter on **Hypothyroidism.** Smoking is not recommended for people who have Raynaud's because it constricts the blood vessels.

In diet, avoid alcohol even though you feel it may be warming to the body; it actually creates a heat loss throughout the body and results in chilling of the extremities. Coffee and caffeine products in over-the-counter pain medications, in chocolate and cola drinks should be avoided because they, too, constrict blood vessels. Be sure you drink enough warm fluids, especially herb teas. Make sure you eat an optimum diet. Plenty of vegetables, moderate fruit, lots of whole grains, nuts, seeds, beans, legumes, fish and chicken.

An important supplement for this condition, besides *iron* when indicated, is *evening primrose oil.* This oil is especially important because one of its properties is to produce, strengthen and maintain the actual membrane of the red blood cell. If this membrane is strong and flexible, then the red cells are able to conform to the shape of the very tiny capillaries at the tips of the fingers and toes. Perhaps Raynaud's is a deficiency of this nutrient. I do not think that there have been any clinical trials of this supplement yet, but theoretically it should help. Gamma linolenic acid, which is the major active ingredient in evening primrose oil, is not found in a typical North American diet. This important nutrient is taken in the dosage of 4 to 6 capsules a day. The only known side effect is headaches in people who are susceptible to alcohol-induced migraines. You can get a headache from the use of evening primrose oil if your liver is toxic or overloaded and not able to process or metabolize either alcohol or oils and fats. If this is the case, read the chapter on **Liver Disease.**

Other helpful supplements include the *B vitamins,* which are important for the nervous system and help the nerves of the fingers; *vitamin E* for thinning the blood and oxygenation; *calcium* and *magnesium* for their effect on cramping; and a good *vitamin* and *mineral* combination.

Rectal Itch

This condition can be caused by food allergies, acidic and spicy foods, Candidiasis or anusitis, an inflammation of the anus. The avoidance of food allergens and the treatment for Candidiasis should be undertaken. If the condition does not completely improve, then there is a treatment with an instrument called Anurex, a cold suppository that is reusable. It is kept in the freezer and inserted into the anus in order to freeze the mucus-forming glands that keep producing an irritating mucus around the anus which can perpetuate this problem of rectal itch. Local creams that can be used would be antifungal medications, *zinc ointment* or *vitamin E oil*. Zinc ointment can be applied in a thick layer and act as a barrier against irritation while the skin is healing. Cortisones should be avoided because they can cause thinning of the skin.

Seborrhea

This condition occurs around the edges of the scalp, over the eyebrows, around the eyes, the lateral corners and to the sides of the nose. It is a flaky, yellowish skin discoloration that sometimes becomes red and bumpy. It is referred to as skin dandruff and is worsened by stress. It responds to treatment with *B vitamins,* 50 mg one to three per day. Skin should also be cleaned with neutral pH soap avoiding either extreme of alkaline or acid. However, the skin would rather be a little more acid, and alkaline soaps tend to dry out the skin, strip the acid mantle and allow irritations and dryness. (Read the chapter **Dry Skin.**)

Shingles

᠅ This is also known as herpes zoster. It is the reactivation of the chickenpox virus, usually in older people and occurring with stress. The treatment is with high doses of *B vitamins,* 50 mg. one to four per day; *vitamin E,* 400 I.U. one to two per day; *B12* injections and acupuncture. At times the pain is so severe that cortisone and strong pain killers must be used so that the person may be able to rest and sleep. The homeopathic remedies for herpes zoster are *Ranunculus* for the neuralgia, *Mezereum* for the itching and burning. *Rhus tox., Apis, Arsenicum, Natrum mur., Cantharis* and *Clematis* have also been used. All these can be used in either 6 to 30c, 4 drops hourly, but the symptoms should be checked in a homeopathic manual.

Sinus Infections

᠅ The sinuses are small cavities in the bones of the head to prevent the skull from being too heavy. The cavities are lined with mucous membranes; these membranes can be irritated or become inflammed and swollen from inhaled or food allergies or from infections. It is important to determine what is allergy and what is infection. With the swelling of the mucous membranes, the channel between the sinus cavities and the nose can become blocked and mucus can build up in the sinuses causing great pressure and considerable pain. The infection starts if there are bacteria trapped in the cavity that can live and grow on the mucus. Temperature and heat identify an acute infection, but sometimes, there is no temperature with a chronic infection.

To treat the chronic condition, try hot compresses on the face or lymphatic massage. (See the chapter on **Edema.**) Avoidance of mucus-forming foods and treatment of allergies is essential. Saline nasal douches are very helpful. Get saline water at a drug store or use a pinch of salt in boiled warm water, hold in a shallow cup under the nostril and inhale gently then blow out. The salt will help constrict the mucus membranes so that the mucus trapped in the sinuses can flow out. Make sure you use a humidifier or a balsam steam inhalation to keep the mucus flowing. Lots of fluid intake is important. My personal favorite for flowing mucus is spicy foods like Szechuan, garlic, curry, or horseradish. A different spice for every day of the week. Exercise also seems to help. The best would be swimming in salt water.

For acute infections, a homeopathic nasal spray called *Euphorbium* can be used as well as hot compresses, shiatsu pressure points around the face and oral homeopathic *Kali bich.* 6c or 30c, which is for tough stringy mucus. For severe and painful sinusitis, *Mercuralis* 6c or 30c, is used by mouth. However, if a bacteria is involved, the above treatments can be used but antibiotic therapy is sometimes necessary. If this is the decided direction, the optimal antibiotic therapy is with *cloxacillin* 250 to 500 mg four times a day for a minimum of two weeks. Less than that amount of time often results in inadequate treatment and continuation and prolongation of symptoms. When on antibiotic therapy, it is important to take acidophilus to replace good bacteria in the intestinal tract that the antibiotics are killing off. A homeopathic remedy can be made from the antibiotic if there are any side effects or if the person feels that the antibiotic remains in the system (See **Making Your Own Remedy**).

Smell and Taste

꙳ These two functions are very much controlled by the mineral zinc. If zinc is lacking in the diet, the taste buds can no longer distinguish the four primary tastes which are sweet, sour, acid and bitter. If a person no longer tastes their food, then the mechanism of feeling satisfied (not necessarily of feeling full) is lost. This can lead to binge eating and overeating. Also, a person will go for more and more sweet foods, again to try to reach some kind of taste satisfaction. I use zinc for people who are binge eaters, sugar cravers or even anorexics or bulimics who don't seem to have a good sense of taste. There is a zinc sulphate hydroxide solution that can be used as a taste test to determine the amount of zinc in the body. This can be administered by a doctor or naturopath. The treatment is to take *zinc picolinate,* 50 mg daily for one month and then 25 mg daily. With prolonged zinc intake, one should also take 1 to 2 mg of *copper* so that copper is not lost from the system.

Smoking

༄ The main point to be made about smoking is to avoid it. The best ways of doing this are outlined in the **Addictions** chapter with homeopathic remedies and herbs as well as acupuncture. There are four points in the ears that can be used to balance the body, by easing irritability and clearing the lungs of the build up of waste material. These can be administered by a doctor trained in ear acupuncture.

Sore Throat

(SEE COLDS AND FLUS)

Sprains

༄ The most common type of sprain is an ankle sprain; however any group of muscles, tendons or ligaments can be strained or sprained. A sprain can be as serious as a broken bone, so it should not be treated lightly. First, an assessment must be made to see if indeed there is a broken bone, then an examination for a torn ligament or tendon.

If you hear a "snap, crackle and pop," you probably have

sprained your ankle. First the tendon snaps from its attachment at the protrusion of the ankle bone at the side, then, if the force is strong enough, it can crack a bit of bone off at the tendon attachment and finally pop it, resulting in a break in the bone. So if you hear something snap, it's important to head for a hospital emergency room where x-rays may be taken. You may be strapped or even put in a cast depending on the severity of sprain. There must be some support to the ankle.

After taking *Arnica* for the trauma, use *Rhus tox.* for the stiffness or *Ruta* if there is more tendon injury to be healed. The dosage is 6c or 30c 4 drops every hour while the pain is severe. Use less as the pain lessens.

Massaging olive oil or castor oil from the toes up to the calf will help clear the swelling. Be sure to use ice for 48 hours, elevate the foot, and stay off it as much as possible. Other strains or sprains can be treated similarly.

Stress

ᑭᎣ Stress today is a favorite media topic. However, without stress of any kind, we would be comatose or sleeping. There must be some stress in our lives to keep us activated. The book *Joy of Stress* by Peter G. Hanson, M.D., does a good job of balancing the positive and negative aspects of stress. In other words, it is not all negative. Stress can be used to cover many definitions of distress in a person's life. If you are overly busy, feel that you are being pulled in many directions and worry that you cannot meet your commitments, then you are, no doubt, under stress.

The best advice for this situation is to set goals and priorities, recognize one's individual limitations, and not overextend oneself. Often good stress counselling will help teach a person how to deal with external causes of stress that are then internalized. Conflicts in personal relationships can also be stress-inducing.

I find that people, particularly women, place too much pressure on themselves to perform in too many roles. They take on a full time job while maintaining a family and caring for both husband and children. Most women feel that they should be able to "do it all" and feel guilty if they can't. The best advice is to cut back on your workload, and to take better care of yourself *before* you become ill and are forced to take time off. Often illness is a subconscious way of cutting back. The issues in allowing oneself to overwork are complex and multiple and it would be wise to sit down with a stress counsellor to work out the conflicts, the sense of self-worth, the goals and priorities, in order to lead a more balanced life.

The best exercise for stress depends on the individual. If someone has a lot of stiffness and tension, they need to do aerobic exercise rather than weight-lifting, which may increase their tension. Someone with a lot of anxiety, panic, and heart racing who has overactive adrenal glands would find tai chi, yoga, walking or swimming more appropriate. Also relaxation tapes would be helpful for this person.

The best supplements for people under stress are the *B vitamins* (the non-yeast brands), 50 mg 2 per day; for anxieties, *niacinamide* 500 mg 2 to 6 per day and *tryptophan* 500 mg, three times a day with 1 or 2 at bedtime to help with sleep. *Tryptophan,* which will soon be available again in the U.S. by prescription, is best used with a carbohydrate drink away from protein by two to three hours. For more recommendations, read the chapters on **Anxiety** and **Insomnia.**

Sunburn

The treatment for sunburn depends on the degree of injury. Above all, do not break any blisters that are forming. Use sunscreen, to prevent future sunburns. If a burn does occur, use *aloe vera gel* or *vitamin A and E creams* immediately and lavishly. Milk of magnesia was recommended by a patient who used it successfully for sunburn. Some people have even used mud or clay to take out the stinging pain of a sunburn. The homeopathic remedies for burns in the chapter on **First Aid** can be taken by mouth.

Surgery

⋙ We will assume your surgery is necessary, that you have received a second and perhaps a third opinion and that the benefits outweigh the risks. Patients who eat an optimum diet and take a basic supplement that includes *zinc, B vitamins, A, D,* and *C, calcium* and *magnesium* before surgery will recover faster. However, it is advisable to avoid the use of *vitamin E,* for 7 to 10 days before surgery, since it is a blood thinner.

Patients are advised to take a Bach Flower Remedy such as *Rescue Remedy* to approach the surgery as calmly as possible. Visualization, relaxation and affirmation tapes are available in your local health food store to help achieve a calm state of mind and to try to influence the subconscious that all will go well during the surgery, that the body will heal rapidly and that health will be restored. Some practitioners of these methods advise patients to visualize the complete hospital stay and all procedures orchestrated to perfection. In the hospital, patients can take *Rescue Remedy* every time they see their doctor and use their battery-powered tape recorders to listen to healing tapes.

After surgery *Phosphorus* 6c is taken, 4 drops for about three doses; this helps clear the anesthetic effects. *Arnica* 30c is taken every 15–60 minutes for pain, shock and swelling. As the pain lessens, the remedy is taken less often. As soon as you are drinking after surgery, *vitamin C* powder can be used in juice or water; 1000 mg every few hours will help healing, help clear the liver of anesthetic, help kidney function and also promote bowel peristalsis. To help bowel function, which is the most important sign watched for after surgery, take a teaspoon of *olive oil* twice per day. When solids are introduced, then the complete range of vitamins can be started. This includes *zinc,* 50 mg per day; *B complex* vitamins, 50 mg twice per day; *vitamin E,* 400 I.U. per day, once the danger of bleeding has passed; and a *multiple vitamin* and *mineral.* For people who have been extremely depleted by their hospitalization or surgery, *blue-green algae,* twice per day and an algae-soy protein drink available in natural food stores could be used for optimum nourishment. The remedy for recovery from surgery is *Veretrum album* 6c, 4 drops three times per day.

Teeth

✍ See the chapter on **Pyorrhea.** Also, read the book by Dr. O. Nara *How to be Dentally Self-Sufficient.* The biggest controversy in dentistry is about mercury amalgam fillings. Sweden has banned mercury fillings, considering them a definite health hazard. More and more people are inquiring about having their amalgams removed. The composites that replace the mercury are a little less stable, may break down a little more easily, and may require earlier replacement. It is best to see a specialist in this work who has spent a lot of time researching the best technique and the best products to use.

When having amalgams removed, be sure to use an oxygen mask during the procedure. Also take extra *vitamin C* before and after removal. Your dentist may advise other supplements. Ear acupuncture in the dental points and relaxation points is very helpful for anesthetic purposes and for faster healing.

Good dental nutrition includes avoidance of sugar and refined foods. With proper brushing and flossing, most cavities can be avoided.

Tendonitis

✍ Tendonitis most commonly occurs at the elbow, as in tennis elbow. But in squash players the overworked tendon is in the wrist. It can be quite debilitating, causing every movement of the arm to be painful.

To prevent tendonitis, first of all, avoid overuse. If the elbow or wrist is starting to hurt, don't push it. Use castor oil packs at night. Put 2 to 3 tablespoons of castor oil, at room temperature, on an old cloth and wrap around the affected area. Tie on with a scarf and wrap in plastic to prevent an oil spill. This often helps to take out the inflammation. Regular icing at the onset of tendonitis or when the area becomes inflamed is helpful. After the tendonitis has cooled down, heat will help. Use a whirlpool, put a heating pad over the castor oil pack, and use hot compresses.

The remedies that help are *Rhus tox.* for stiffness and *Ruta,* which is specifically for tendons. The dosage is 6c or 30c, 4 drops every two hours for acute pain and less for less severe pain.

Acupuncture can often help this condition. Medically, physiotherapy is prescribed and ultrasound is used. Chiropractors use ultrasound and sometimes adjust the area; some also use acupuncture.

Travelling Advice

&. Travel light is the best tip and this includes your nutritional supplements. If you need to take them with you, use a combined *multiple vitamin and mineral* to try to eliminate many bottles. For preventing diarrhea, take *hydrochloric acid tablets* (unless you have an ulcer), 1 to 2 at the end of each meal to kill off any indigenous parasites. The old saying is that you may be used to the bugs in your own home town but not the critters elsewhere. Take *acidophilus* to build up the good bacteria in your intestines once or twice a day. There is now a liquid on the market which does not have to be refrigerated.

Prevention

Do not drink the water; this means ice, fruit drinks and milk shakes.

Do not eat salads or cut fruits, except fruits you peel yourself.

Eat only freshly cooked food.

Drink boiled water, commercially bottled water or mineral water.

Dry foods are usually safe.

Wash your hands often.

Think about everything that you ingest, even the water for brushing your teeth.

Treatment

Use dietary treatment first. Antibiotic or antidiarrheal pills can be dangerous and actually prolong the illness.

The first day, drink only clear fluids: soups, juices, teas.

The second day, eat only rice, apple sauce, and bananas.

The third day, add dry bland foods, nothing greasy, fried or spicy.

By the fourth day you should be able to move up to a normal diet but do so slowly.

Avoid dairy and citrus for at least a week.

If your bowels loosen at any time, move back to clear fluids.

Go to the nearest doctor or hospital

If any symptom stays on for more than five to six days.

If fever, bloody diarrhea, or vomiting and diarrhea occur together. Dehydration occurs when vomiting and diarrhea are present. Watch your urine output.

Warning

Antidiarrheal pills should be used only to control diarrhea for short periods of time when absolutely necessary, such as long road trips.

Antibiotics can be dangerous when used for diarrhea and should be prescribed by a doctor. They can lead to overgrowth of Candida in the intestines. (Read the chapter on **Candidiasis.**)

Watch young children with diarrhea; they dehydrate faster. They can go without food but don't let them go without fluids. Warm baths can help to rehydrate.

Read the chapters on **Diarrhea, Gas** and **Digestion** for further tips on symptoms that continue after a bout of travellers' diarrhea.

Ulcers

Over the years there have been many different theories on the cause of ulcers and as many different treatments. The current controversy is whether or not ulcers could have a infective basis. An organism called campylobacter causes infection and ulceration of the stomach lining. If people have an ulceration due to campylobacter, then the organism has to be killed before the ulcer can heal. There is an antibody test to determine if a person has this infection. Gastroscopy, looking into the stomach with a fiberoptic scope, can also include a biopsy of the stomach to identify an infection or other abnormalities. If campylobacter is found, *Pepto Bismol* may be the cure. It is now being researched. Ask your doctor. Investigation by barium swallow will identify an ulceration and the usual antacid treatments are instituted.

A diet for ulcers used to be a low fiber bland diet but the best diet advice is to individually observe what makes the pain worse and what makes the pain better. Smoking and alcohol certainly are contraindicated for people with ulcers. Milk may cause problems by increasing stomach acid. Antacids and ulcer medications might themselves cause problems in the long run since they interfere with food digestion. Cabbage juice (use young cabbages), 4 ounces per day, helps ulcers with a constituent that has been labeled vitamin U.

Supplements that may help heal the ulcers are *B vitamins,* 50 mg 1 to 2 per day; *zinc,* 25 mg daily; *vitamin A,* 10,000 I.U. 1 to 2 a day; and herbs such as *comfrey, slippery elm* and *aloe vera.* Homeopathic *Nux vomica* and *Lycopodium* are often used to treat ulcers in a person with constitutional characteristics of those remedies. The usual dosage is 4 drops, three times per day. (Read about these two remedies in the **Remedy** section of this book.)

Vaginitis

℘ Vaginitis is most often due to yeast overgrowth rather than bacterial overgrowth. The diagnosis is made clinically, especially in the case of yeast, and confirmed by vaginal swab although the positive yield of yeast identification in a laboratory is often low. Doctors often must go by the clinical impression plus the history; that is, vaginitis prior to the period, worse after overindulgence in sweets, bread or fruit, white cheesy, itchy, irritating discharge and also a history of being on birth control pills and antibiotics. A bacterial vaginitis can usually be diagnosed by a swab. If it is a common Gardnerella, Strep or Hemophilus and on internal exam the infection is not in the fallopian tubes and there are no fever or chills, then a local douche with Betadine is often acceptable. If the bacterial infection is Gonorrhea or Chlamydia, then the treatment is with oral antibiotics. Remember to take *acidophilus* with the antibiotic to prevent yeast infection.

To prevent yeast vaginitis, avoid tight jeans and wear loose cotton underwear (which may have to be boiled or ironed to kill all the yeast spores). Be aware that acidifying spermicides can irritate the vagina and encourage yeast overgrowth.

Don't wipe with scented or dyed toilet paper and don't use scented or deodorized pads or tampons. Make sure tampons themselves are not the cause of your symptoms. Or alternate between pads and tampons. Be sure your partner is not passing yeast back to you during intercourse; use a condom. Natural douches include baking soda or vinegar (1 tablespoon to 2 cups of water), *acidophilus* or *yogurt*.

Treatment for yeast vaginitis is often given locally. In some cases, this may be enough to provide symptomatic relief. However, if the condition is persistent, it must be treated on a broader scale with diet, *acidophilus* by mouth, *acidophilus* mixed with yogurt to make a paste which can be used vaginally, and sometimes oral antifungal medications. (Please see the chapter on **Candidiasis.**)

Varicose Veins

⏳ Varicose veins are due to weak valves in the veins of the legs which are unable to push the blood away from the legs against the force of gravity. This results in swollen veins which can cause pain and disfigurement. Although this condition is often hereditary, some natural remedies and recommendations can help reduce the extent of the condition. One must avoid obesity and constipation. The diet must be high fiber in content and exercise is essential to improve circulation. Elevate the legs, wear support hose, lie on a slant board for several minutes a day.

The nutrients that will aid this condition are *bioflavins,* part of the vitamin C complex that heal veins and capillaries, 500 to 1000 mg per day; *witch hazel* used as a compress on very swollen veins; homeopathic drops of *Hamamelis* 6 or 30c, 4 drops three times a day.

A process called sclerotherapy, which is the injection of small veins with saline to collapse them, can remove unsightly veins.

Some specialists claim that this can be done for any size of varicosity.

Warts

🔊 Warts on the fingers or warts on the soles of the feet can be treated using *castor oil, vitamin E, vitamin A, aloe vera* or *tea tree oil*. Any one of them can be applied directly to the wart, covered with a Band-Aid and worn each night. A person afflicted might try one or more of these treatments but results often take several weeks. As the callous over the root of the viral wart is removed, little black dots will be seen. This is the virus itself and, when it is exposed to air, it often begins to die. This is often a more convenient way of treating warts than going to a dermatologist to have a burning, cutting or acid treatment administered.

X-rays

🔊 X-rays are sometimes necessary, although often overused. It is a tool that doctors depend heavily on and find hard to let go of even in the face of evidence that they may be harmful. The best recommendation is to question the necessity of the x-rays before receiving them.

Next read Dr. Rosalie Bertell's book *No Immediate Danger*. She heads The International Institute of Concern for Public Health. Dr. Bertell's book describes the dangers of even small amounts of radiation. If x-rays are essential, lessen the side effects with an x-ray homeopathic remedy, available from your homeopathic doctor.

REMEDIES

Homeopathic and Herbal Remedies for Home Use

᳍ Homeopathy has been practiced for 200 years. It is the science of using extremely low potency substances to cure illness. It seems to enhance the natural healing ability of the body. It does not suppress or overwhelm the human being behind the illness.

The dosage for acute illness is usually 6C given every one to four hours depending on the severity of the condition. The worse the illness, the more often the remedy is repeated. The higher potencies, such as 200C, are used in general to treat for emotional balance and constitutional balance. They can be used by a homeopath for severe disease in the acute stage.

The general rule for the use of a remedy is that if it has not caused a change in the condition after six to eight doses, then the remedy should be stopped, the case history of the patient should be taken again and a more appropriate remedy started. Or a homeopath should be consulted.

It is important not to use coffee, mints, camphor, chamomile herb or chemicals with strong odors during the time of homeopathic treatment. All these substances will antidote the remedies.

Please be advised that you should not allow your remedies to go through the x-ray at airports. This will antidote them. Have the attendant walk them around the x-ray equipment as you would with your camera film.

The references for this materia medica are:

Materia Medica with Repertory by William Boericke, M.D.
Everybody's Guide to Homeopathic Medicines by Stephen Cummings and Dana Ullman.
Homeopathy at Home by Trevor Smith, M.D.
Homeopathy for the First Aider by Dorothy Sheppard, M.D.

Aconite

THE KEYNOTE OF THIS REMEDY IS SUDDENNESS OF ONSET.

For the very first signs of a cold or flu, especially when brought on by an exposure to cold weather. For asthma, dry suffocating cough, sore throat and high temperature with great thirst. For tonsillitis, teething and toothache. For animal bites, sleeplessness, intolerance of pain, stiff neck and ringing ears. For menstrual periods suppressed or delayed due to worry or fear. For abdominal pain which is made worse by drinking cold water. For great pain; if the condition (whatever it might be) is so severe you don't know what to give, use aconite first. Symptoms are sudden, violent and brief.

For extreme emotions, fear, grief, anxiety and restlessness, a sense of impending doom and bereavement. Aconite may be used for the fear of surgery or dental work. There is also fear of crowds. These intense emotions may accompany the physical symptoms. The appearance will be of fear and restlessness; one cheek may be flushed and one pale. This is unlike Belladonna which has both cheeks flushed and more delirium than wide-awake fear.

Symptoms are worse at midnight, when lying on affected side, in a warm room, from tobacco smoke, in cold dry winds and listening to music.

Symptoms are better in the open air, with perspiring and with the bedclothes thrown off.

Aethusa

ᦉ For milk intolerance especially for babies with colic.

Apis

THE KEYNOTES ARE A BEE STING PAIN AND HIVE-LIKE SWELLING.

ᦉ For burning or stinging pains where flushing, swelling or puffing occurs. Especially good for swelling of the lower eyelid which looks like a bag of water. Symptoms mostly on the right side. For acute allergic reactions, edema, bee stings, hives, nettle rash, acute kidney infections, and right sided ovarian cysts. For synovitis, swollen gums, incontinence in older people, shingles, teething, sore throat, tonsillitis and infected nailbed. There is no thirst. There is listlessness and lack of concentration.

Emotionally the person may be sad, depressed, tearful or irritable and suspicious. He may try to avoid medical attention.

Symptoms are worse from getting wet, during late afternoon, after sleeping, from heat in any form, when touched and when in a closed and heated room.

Symptoms are better from a change of position or walking about in the open air and from cold.

Arnica

THE KEYNOTE IS FOR ANY INJURY, EMOTIONAL OR
PHYSICAL.

ᴥ The number one remedy for pain, shock, swelling, bruising
after any injury or surgery, including dental work and childbirth. This can be taken at any time after the injury no matter
how remote, if there are still symptoms. Arnica cream can be
applied directly on the injured part. If the wound is open or the
skin is broken, the cream must not be used because it will cause
the wound to fester. Also good for mental as well as physical
shock. For bruises, sprains, physical exhaustion, sleeplessness
due to over-exhaustion. For gout, with a fear of being touched,
loss of voice, toothache and bee or wasp stings. Other classic
symptoms include: the bed feels too hard, a fear of being
touched or approached, the whole body feels beaten up and
bruised, muscles feel achy.

Symptoms worse from touch, from exposure to hot sun, from
motion and in damp, cold conditions.

Symptoms better when lying down with the head low and
not propped up.

Arsenicum Album

THE KEYNOTES ARE ANXIETY AND FEAR.

ᴥ No matter what the physical illness may be, if there is great
fear, restlessness and anxiety with weakness, exhaustion, shud-
dering chills and burning pains which are worse at night, then
this is the remedy of choice. The weakness and exhaustion seem
exaggerated but it becomes evident that the person's restlessness
and agitation is wearing them out. The patient is terrified of

illness, fearful of death, and expresses great insecurity, which, of course, makes things all the worse. The patient is extremely meticulous and everything must be perfectly clean and tidy. There is a fear of being alone but also a fear of being observed closely which borders on paranoia. The body feels cold and chilled and desires hot drinks in spite of the burning nature of the pains.

For vomiting and diarrhea caused by eating bad meat, fruit or vegetables, can't bear the sight or smell of food. May feel they have been poisoned. Good for children with upset stomaches from food with burning pain. For asthma, worse at 2 a.m. with anxiety. For any pain which is burning and better with heat. For sore throat which burns but is better with sips of hot liquids. For eye pain or infection which is better with hot cloths. For psoriasis, thrush, tough mucus, and hay fever. For burning vaginitis which is better with hot water washes.

Symptoms worse after midnight to 3 a.m. and between 1–2 p.m. Worse at the ocean and from cold and wet weather.

Symptoms better by keeping warm, with cool air around the head, from warm or hot drinks taken in sips, and from company.

Belladonna

THE KEYNOTES ARE HOT, RED, THROBBING, INFLAMMATION.

꼉 The patient looks flushed and feverish and dull with dilated pupils and bright red dry skin. The fever is high, the onset is acute and the pain is severe, throbbing and burning. The fever may go very high and lead to hallucinations and even destructive behavior.

For colds, earaches or any condition with sudden onset and flushing, throbbing heat with blood rushing to the area. Menopausal hot flushes, menstrual pains, infections, boils or headaches. The headache has a characteristic band-like pressure feeling. The hollow areas of the body may feel the sensation of a ball inside. For swollen glands, swollen joints, facial neuralgia, chickenpox, sunstroke, measles, air sickness. Menstrual periods are early and heavy. For mumps, bladder infections, sore throat and tonsillitis. For loss of voice, toothache and teething, stiff neck and incontinence.

Symptoms are worse in the afternoon and at night, from noise, from lying down, from bright light, from touch, and from jarring movement.

Symptoms are better from warmth and while lying down, especially on the abdomen.

Bryonia

THE KEYNOTE IS WORSE FROM MOVEMENT.

᪣ The movement can be from walking, moving the eyes, even swallowing. Deep breathing, talking or laughing can bring on a painful coughing spell.

The patient is irritable, gets angry easily, hates interrogation and wants to be left alone. The patient may feel confused and appear dim-witted.

For tearing and stitching pains which are worse from moving and better from resting.

For respiratory conditions where colds go down into the chest, with dry painful cough which can be violent i.e., bronchitis; there is dryness of the air passages, dry lips, tongue and throat and excessive thirst, especially for cold drinks. With bryonia colds and flus there are joint and muscle aches, which are worse with movement. For digestive disorders, food lies like a weight in the stomach, stomach is too painful to touch and worse with any movement. The abdomen may be painfully distended with gas. For diarrhea after eating over-ripe fruit, or drinking cold water when overheated or feverish. The stool is usually dry and hard. For musculoskeletal problems like lumbago, painful knee joints, painful hip joints, rheumatism, gout and stiff neck.

There may be food cravings for milk, sweets or sour fruits. The patient is thirsty for large amounts of liquids.

Symptoms are worse from movement, from warmth, in the summer, from eating fruit, bread, beans or milk. Symptoms are worse on the right side of the body.

Symptoms are better from lying completely still, in cool weather, from cold applications and firm pressure.

Calc. Carb.

THE KEYNOTES ARE OVERWORK AND OVERWORRY.

This remedy is used for some acute conditions but it is mostly a constitutional remedy which means it is used to boost a person's vital force. When a chubby, sweaty child has a minor complaint, this remedy can be used to help them get over it. The person may be physically and mentally weak or tired. The body is flabby with poor muscle tone and tiredness and the sweat is profuse and sour smelling. Dislikes milk, coffee, tobacco and hot food. Craves eggs, wine, salt or sweets. Tendency to feel the cold and catch cold easily, and has cold damp feet and clammy hands.

Treats symptoms of cracked skin, premenstrual tensions, warts and obesity or any minor complaint in which *Calc carb* is the known constitutional remedy.

Symptoms worse from cold air and draughts, in damp weather, at night and from standing. Worse from exertion and fright.

Symptoms better in dry weather, from warmth (but not the sun) and while lying on the painful side.

Calendula

🙝 Available as a tincture or a cream. As a tincture, it is a useful antiseptic and analgesic. It is used to clean wounds and pack wounds. Ten drops in a few ounces of water is the usual dosage. The gauze that is used to pack a wound can be moistened with dilute tincture. As a cream it is used for any skin eczema. Unlike cortisone creams, which suppress symptoms and drive the condition deeper into the body, calendula heals from the inside out.

Cantharis

THE KEYNOTE IS SEVERE BURNING PAIN.

🙝 For local irritations with pain which is burning and raw. For burns and scalds before blisters form, for sunburn or for burning pain in the bladder before, during and after passing urine. Urine scalds and is passed drop by drop; there is a constant and intolerable urge to urinate.

Symptoms are worse from touch, while passing urine and after drinking cold water or coffee.

Symptoms are better after belching or passing gas.

Carbo. Veg.

THE KEYNOTES ARE PALE AND PULSELESS.

🙝 For mild food poisoning especially when caused by fish. For heartburn with excessive gas. For varicose veins and ulcers, hoarseness, rough throat without pain and loss of voice. Also for hypertensive, shock-like states and in chronic emphysema.

Symptoms are worse after eating fatty foods, during cold, damp, frosty weather, in the evening and at night.

Symptoms are better on passing gas, being fanned and after sleep.

Chamomilla

THE KEYNOTE IS EXTREME IRRITABILITY.

With this remedy there is pain and one does not know what to do with it. There is fretfulness, fussiness, irritability, impatience and whining. Children are treated more with this remedy than adults probably because adults learn to control their irritability. Nothing pleases and everything bothers these patients. They immediately reject what they just demanded and a temper tantrum can ensue. Their pain can be from teething, wisdom teeth, painful periods, headaches. The face is flushed with one cheek red and the other white and they are thirsty.

Symptoms are worse in a warm bed, eating warm food at night, with touch, with any demands, open air, wind and cold.

Symptoms are better with constant motion and rocking, with cold cloths and fasting.

Dulcamara

THE KEYNOTES ARE COLD AND DAMP.

For colds and flus occurring on cold, damp, wet nights toward the close of summer. Nose and eyes streaming. Nasal discharge excessive in warm rooms, yet stuffed up when outside. Nose can become sore from the constant running and blowing.

Echinacea

᷼ A tincture. This is an herbal remedy noted for its natural antibiotic properties. For any infection, especially colds and flus it is used 10 drops in 4 ounces of water three or four times a day. For the prevention of colds in a susceptible person, 10 drops each morning is very useful. People with Epstein-Barr virus use this remedy as a preventive.

Euphrasia

᷼ A tincture. This herb is called eyebright. It is used specifically for eye washes. For tiredness and minor infections, styes and irritations, put two to three drops in an eyecup with sterile water and bathe the eye several times a day. However, do not treat eye infections without the advice of your doctor. (See the chapter on **Eyes.**)

Ferrum Phos.

THE KEYNOTE IS ACUTE INFLAMMATION.

᷼ For the first stage of acute inflammation and early colds, flus, and earaches, especially before specific symptoms start. The onset of symptoms may not be as sudden or dramatic as with *Aconite* or *Belladonna* and may come after overexertion. The patient is exhausted but still alert, unlike *Belladonna* where the patient is dull and stuporous. For headache with a hot red face and vomiting relieved by nosebleeds. For nosebleeds with no other symptoms.

The person is flushed and hot with fever. The face is red with circular patches. The person is excitable and talkative. The appetite varies greatly from insatiable hunger to total loss of appetite. The person cannot tolerate the hair being touched. Symptoms are worse at night, from cold and from touch.

Symptoms are better in summer, from warmth, from cold applications, while walking slowly, and from gentle motion.

Gelsemium

THE KEYNOTES ARE EXHAUSTION LEADING TO FLU.

For the treatment of influenza and influenza-like colds. For sneezing, sore throat, flushing, aching, trembling, heavy eyes, weary and heavy aching muscles, difficulty in swallowing, runny nose, dizziness and chills running down the back. The patient is mentally and physically weak and drowsy and avoids movement because of exhaustion. Every part of the body feels weak and heavy. Headache is throbbing and spreads from the base of the neck to the forehead above the eyes and feels like a tight band. For mental exhaustion, writer's cramp, neuralgia and sunstroke. Also for treatment of anticipation anxiety, i.e., pre-game or pre-exam nerves. There is absence of thirst even with a high temperature.

Symptoms worse from sudden fright, excessive excitement, bad news, frustration and anticipation. Worse when exposed to direct sunlight, in a hot room, before a thunderstorm and in cold damp weather. Worse around 10 a.m. worse with movement but movement helps muscular pains.

Symptoms better in the open air, from continued movement, from alcoholic stimulants, after sweating and after passing large amounts of pale urine.

Hepar Sulph.

THE KEYNOTES ARE HYPERSENSITIVITY AND IRRITABILITY.

ᐯ These patients are extremely sensitive to touch, cold and pain in the affected or infected part. This is the most sensitive remedy to the cold. Even a slight draft on part of the body can bring on symptoms. These patients also seem to overreact to pain and may faint with pain. They are also extremely cross and irritable, get angry at the slightest thing and, although they may become violent, they do not hit out like a child who needs *Chamomilla*. The smells of sweat and discharges are sour and offensive, and are profuse, thick, yellow or cheesy. This type of patient likes sour, spicy, strong-tasting foods. There may be a dislike of fats and a strong thirst.

For croupy cough after exposure to cold, dry air, with rattling in the chest but little mucus. For sore throat with the sensation of a splinter or fishbone in the throat. For earache with offensive discharge, and for chronic tonsillitis especially when associated with a hearing loss; also for sinusitis. For injuries which tend to become infected and are very painful. For boils that are exquisitely sensitive to touch, worse with cold applications and with offensive pus when they come to a head. The skin is generally unhealthy, sweaty and sensitive.

Symptoms are worse in cold air, cold dry winds and drafts, in the winter, in the evening after midnight, when the head is uncovered and lying on the painful side; with motion, exertion, and wearing tight clothing.

Symptoms are better from warmth, from wrapping up, (especially the head), after a meal, and in warm wet weather.

Hypericum

THE KEYNOTE IS NERVE PAIN.

꙳ For nerve injury, especially to the fingers and toes and coccyx, and for puncture wounds. Pain is severe. For injuries by cat bite and sharp objects, spinal injuries, headache with a floating sensation as a result of a fall. For blows on fingers or toes.

Symptoms worse from cold and damp especially before a storm, from touch, from 6 p.m. to 10 p.m. and in the dark.

Symptoms better while bending head backwards and while keeping still. Hypericum tincture is used as an analgesic and antiseptic for washing out wounds or soaking or packing wounds.

Ignatia

THE KEYNOTES ARE FRUSTRATION AND GRIEF.

꙳ This remedy is excellent for treating the ill effects of grief or worry. It is mostly a mental, emotional or constitutional remedy. It is used for shock and fear and grief after the death of a loved one. It is especially useful for postpartum depression when the new mother is overwhelmed with all her extra responsibilities and wants to be the most perfect mother but finds it impossible to do everything. She can then become stricken with fear and worry and approach hysteria with her frustration.

Ignatia patients never cry in public but they do give away their feelings by loud frequent sighs. They do not like to be criticized but tend to be very self-critical and perfectionistic. There is usually a strong dislike of tobacco smoke approaching fanaticism.

It is also used for throbbing headaches and sciatica. Or it is used for any condition that was brought on by grief, fear, anger, embarrassment or humiliation. There can be insomnia from the emotional strain, the feeling of a lump in the throat from repressed feelings or symptoms of nervous exhaustion. Symptoms seem contradictory. There is nausea relieved by eating; heavy foods are digested better then light foods, yet hunger is made more intense by eating.

Symptoms worse in the morning, from cold, from eating sweets, coffee or alcohol, from tobacco smoke, and from suppressing grief.

Symptoms better while eating and from moving to a new position.

Ipecac

THE KEYNOTE IS PERSISTENT VOMITING.

For persistent and continuous nausea and vomiting as in morning sickness, motion sickness or food poisoning. The vomiting may not even relieve the nausea temporarily. The situation is made worse by the smell of food and can be due to eating too rich a meal. Vomiting is worse after eating or drinking. There is surprisingly little thirst and not the anxiety and chilliness seen in *Arsenicum*. There may be much mucus vomited and this makes it a remedy for bronchitis with vomiting. There can be a greenish type of diarrhea with gas and abdominal cramps. The tongue may be clean and uncoated, and salivation accompanies the feeling of inevitable vomiting.

Symptoms worse when lying down, in cold weather, and after eating veal or pork.

Symptoms better when at rest, with eyes closed, and out in the open.

Kali Bich.

THE KEYNOTE IS TOUGH, STICKY, GLUEY, STRINGY MUCUS.

This remedy is for acute or particular symptoms and does not have many mental or emotional signs except for irritability and indifference.

For symptoms brought on by a change from cold to hot weather. For catarrh with a stringy discharge from sinusitis, sore throat, eye infection or ear infection. For migraines with blurred vision before headache, and sinus headaches. Pains move rapidly and are limited to small areas of the body. Symptoms alternate between joint pains, digestive problems, respiratory illness and diarrhea.

Symptoms worse in the morning, especially 2 to 3 a.m., from alcohol, during hot weather. Hot weather can worsen arthritic conditions.

Symptoms better from heat and a warm bed.

Ledum

THE KEYNOTE IS PUNCTURES.

◈ This remedy is used for all puncture wounds from claws, stingers, needles, nails and knives. The type of injury is more cold and red and throbbing than a *Belladonna* injury which is hot and red and throbbing. However, it is relieved by cold applications. It will also treat black eyes and bad bruising that feels cold and is better with cold applications.

Lycopodium

THE KEYNOTES ARE RIGHT-SIDEDNESS AND INSECURITY.

◈ This is a constitutional remedy which is used more for chronic conditions. Therefore, the general mental and emotional characteristics should be sought for the proper prescription. Lycopodium people are insecure and afraid, like the cowardly lion in The Wizard of Oz. They are afraid to try new things and fearful in public situations. There is a fear of rejection and criticism. They may give a front of courage like the lion and intimidate younger and weaker people. They may have many fears; of death, the dark, of crowds. Their symptoms tend to be in the digestive system, the nervous system, the bladder and the respiratory system.

The remedy can be used for premenstrual tension and irritability relieved when the period starts. For cystitis, when passing large amounts of pale urine, sometimes with a sediment. For digestive symptoms such as heartburn; craving for sweet foods which then cause indigestion, gas, and bloating; hiccoughs with acidity and bloating; excessive hunger which is satisfied easily; and abdominal pain which is worse with tight clothing. Hunger may wake them at night, or there maybe headaches when skipping meals as in hypoglycemia. Treats anticipatory fear of failure. For coldness in one foot; for symptoms or pains which are definitely worse on the right side or begin on the right side and move to the left. For tonsillitis, sore throats and colds, worse on the right side. These people dislike exercise; they prefer to be alone, but with someone nearby.

Symptoms worse between 4 and 8 p.m. Bad tempered on waking, worse in stuffy rooms, from cold air, cold food or liquid, when hurried or worried. Foods which may aggravate the condition are meat, oysters, onions, cabbage and milk.

Symptoms better after warm drinks, midnight, on loosening clothing around the abdomen, in cold fresh air, and when occupied.

Nux Vomica

THE KEYNOTES ARE TYPE-A PERSONALITY AND HANGOVERS.

⁓ This is a constitutional remedy prescribed more for the mental and emotional symptoms.

This individual is impatient, irritable, tense, overanxious and on edge, oversensitive to noise, odors, bright light and music. This could describe a person with a hangover and a Type-A personality. These people are also driven to overwork and are impatient and demanding with others. Insomnia is common due to the sensitivity to noise and the overactive mind and they may wake early. They are very irritable if woken from a nap. They are very orderly and fussy. They are chilly and are worse in cold, dry weather. If there is a fever they get chills and are unable to keep warm. There is a craving for fats, milk and spicy foods.

For the ill effects of over-eating, or indulging in coffee, smoking, alcohol or drugs. This craving for stimulants maybe an attempt to keep the mind activated to continue working. For multiple digestive complaints of heartburn two to three hours after eating, abdominal pain, gas, bloating, nausea, constipation, diarrhea, or burning and itching hemorrhoids. For the treatment of morning sickness, insomnia, travel sickness with vomiting from the least motion, if the psychological picture also fits. For stuffy colds and asthma. In a true *Nux vomica* individual, respiratory symptoms are accompanied by digestive disturbances. There is a painful but ineffectual urge to urinate, which is part of the tendency to muscle spasms and twitching. There are low back pain and a stiff neck and headaches from the muscle tension symptoms.

Symptoms are worse between 3 and 4 a.m. on waking in the morning, and from cold, dry, windy weather. They are worse with mental overwork and anger and from overeating.

Symptoms are better in the evening, from being covered, and from warmth and sleep.

Pulsatilla

THE KEYNOTES ARE WEEPYNESS AND CHANGEABILITY.

ଉ This is a constitutional remedy which means it is useful for many conditions and often prescribed for the mental and emotional symptoms. Pulsitilla people are gentle, soft, and sensitive. They like the attention of others and want to be liked; they seek approval. They can be weepy and vulnerable and need to be comforted and consoled. They may be afraid of being alone and afraid of the dark. Their moods change quickly; they are weepy one moment and happy and laughing the next. They cry easily from a criticism or a perceived insult or even from thinking of something sad or overhearing an argument. They pity themselves when they get sick and wonder "why does this have to happen to me?" They are warm-blooded and like the cold. They do not like heat or warm rooms and become lethargic. They change their minds frequently, cannot make a decision, and are easily swayed.

Pulsitilla is used for any mucusy condition with yellow-green thick discharge; hayfever, styes on the eyelids, conjunctivitis with thick yellow discharge, mumps with swollen glands, measles, sinusitis with yellow discharge. For menopause, menstrual pain with nausea and vomiting, for suppressed, delayed or irregular periods. For premenstrual tension with weepiness and loneliness, the individual can change to the opposite mood quickly and be angry and strident. For cystitis with urinary frequency, pain and distress. For joint inflammation with swelling or redness and the pain jumps from joint to joint. There are digestive disturbances with bloating and sensitivity of the abdomen after eating. There is an aversion to fat or greasy food, but there is a craving for these foods which bring on the symptoms. There is an absence of thirst and rapid change in symptoms.

Symptoms are worse in the evening before midnight, from heat, humidity, after rich foods such as fat, pork, meat, milk and bread. Worse from being chilled when hot.

Symptoms are better in the open air, from cold cloths and cold food and drinks, while lying on the painful side and from being uncovered.

Rhus Tox.

THE KEYNOTES ARE IMPROVEMENT WITH MOVEMENT, WORSENING WITH REST.

๛ This remedy is made from poison ivy so it treats contact with this plant.

This is a useful remedy for sprains and strains of joints, tendons or ligaments. The pain is usually worse at the first movement but gets better with continued movement. The joints are stiff, swollen and painful, which is made worse by cold applications and better by heat and by pressure. The cause is usually overexertion and worry in people who are restless and cannot sit still. It is used for treating conditions accompanied by rashes. Also it is used for symptoms after surgery; for sciatica, pain in ligaments, a stiff neck and rheumatism. For chickenpox, poison ivy, shingles, eczema and cold sores where the lesions are itchy and burning at night. For a tickling cough with thirst and achiness of joints, which are worse at rest and better with movement. Anxiety and restlessness accompany most symptoms with inability to sit still due to impatience, worry or pain. They are sleepless from the mental and physical restlessness. The body is chilly and worse in cold and damp weather. There is thirst for cold drinks or milk but the cold may aggravate the condition.

Symptoms are worse at the beginning of movement, during rest, from overexertion, from cold and wet weather and after midnight.

Symptoms are better during warm weather, with gentle movement and from warm applications.

Sepia

THE KEYNOTES ARE SLUGGISHNESS, HEAVINESS AND ANGER.

∂ This is a constitutional remedy best known as a female remedy for hormone balancing. There is no energy and a cold, withdrawn, apathetic attitude. But if the person can be motivated to move or exercise, the energy comes back and they feel better on all levels. They may be sad and weepy one moment but angry and spiteful the next. They dislike consolation and push people away but do not like to be alone. They have an aversion to food and the smell of food. They may feel hungry, but eating does not satisfy them. They are often constipated and crave sour, bitter and spicy foods. They dislike fat, bread, milk, meat and salt. There is a peculiar symptom of the sensation of a ball in the throat, abdomen, rectum or uterus. There is also a pressure or bearing-down pain from the uterus and a tendency to keep the legs crossed, which is a keynote.

Sepia suits dark women with sallow skin who have the following symptoms: Indifference to loved ones yet sad and fearful of being left alone, irritability and anger. It treats premenstrual tension with pain and delayed periods. For menopausal hot flushes with fainting and hot sweats from the slightest exertion. There are also ulcers, warts and urinary incontinence.

Symptoms are worse in the afternoon and evening at 4 to 6 p.m., with the cold, with consolation, from tobacco smoke and before a storm. Worse eating fat, bread, milk, meat or sour foods.

Symptoms are better in a warm bed, from heat, and after dancing.

Staphasagria

THE KEYNOTE IS VULNERABILITY.

This is another constitutional remedy. It suits a person who has been treated with disrespect and remains vulnerable. It is therefore prescribed in a high potency for strengthening a person's vital force but as an acute remedy in this context we will look at it for one main purpose. It is an excellent remedy for bladder irritation after intercourse or after cystoscopy examination of the bladder or any prostate surgery. (See the chapter on **Bladder Infection**.)

Thuja

THE KEYNOTE IS WARTS AND GROWTHS.

 This is a very useful remedy for treating warts of any description and for the after-effects of immunization. It is also used for headaches in the morning on waking and which are aggravated by sleeping; for pain at the end of urination that cuts like a knife; and for sleeplessness.

Symptoms are worse from cold and damp, at night from the heat of the bed at 3 a.m. and 3 p.m. and after breakfast.

Symptoms are better after sweating, from scratching or being massaged and after stretching the extremities.

Urtica Urens

THE KEYNOTE IS RAISED RED SWELLINGS.

 This remedy is made from the stinging nettle plant and it treats the type of symptoms that contact with this plant will cause. Raised red swellings that are intensely itchy, such as hives, are treated. They are usually made worse by warmth and exercise and better with cold applications and by lying still. This is also an acute remedy for burns and scalds. It is used internally until the symptoms of pain abate.

How to Make Your Own Remedy

 Homeopathic pharmacies make up remedies from scratch. They take a substance and dilute it to the correct potency for a particular use. However, in an emergency, you can make your own remedy. This might be when someone has taken a medication but can't seem to get rid of the side effects. This is not meant to treat serious or life-threatening side effects or proven allergies to drugs.

The method is to take one unit of the substance, a pill or a teaspoon of liquid; crush the pill to a fine powder. Then dissolve it in 3 ounces of pure distilled water in a small bottle with a cap. Pound the bottle hard against the palm of your hand or on a hard pillow 50 times. Take 1 tsp. of the liquid from that bottle and put it into a second bottle with 3 ounces of water and pound that bottle 50 times. Rinse out the first bottle well and put 1 tsp. of the new mixture into 3 ounces of water and pound it 50 times. Do this procedure back and forth six times and you will have diluted the drug so that it has no chemical action but you have imprinted the remedy into the water. This imprinted water can have the effect of removing any residual drug from the body. The last 3 ounces can be kept in the fridge and used, 1 tsp. two to three times a day until the symptoms are gone or for a few weeks. To preserve the remedy, use one part vodka or other potable alcohol and 4 parts water. The alcohol prevents bacteria from growing in the water.

To illustrate the effectiveness of this treatment, consider a study done with rats who were given arsenic. After the rats stopped excreting arsenic in their urine, one-half of the rats were given homeopathic arsenic. Those rats started excreting arsenic into the urine again. So there was arsenic still in the body; it is stored in the fat cells and the remedy helped get rid of it.

In fact all the drugs we have taken in our lifetimes have the potential to still be in our bodies. We have all heard the stories about people who go on long fasts who say that they can taste old medicines that they had dozens of years ago.

SYMPTOMS AND REMEDIES:
A QUICK REFERENCE GUIDE

ᕽ There are thousands of homeopathic remedies. This listing gives only those remedies for the complaints and conditions that are listed in this book. The following remedies are the most widely used in my practice.

TIMING OF SYMPTOMS	REMEDIES
Morning	Nux vomica, Thuja
Mid-morning	Sepia
Afternoon	Belladonna, Sepia
3 P.M.	Thuja
4 P.M.–8P.M.	Lycopodium
6 P.M.	Hypericum
Evening	Carbo veg., Pulsatilla, Sepia
Midnight	Arsenicum, Rhus tox.
Night	Ferrum phos.
2 A.M.	Arsenicum
2 A.M.–5 A.M.	Kali bich.
3 A.M.–4 A.M.	Nux vomica, Thuja

SYMPTOMS	REMEDIES
Abdominal pain	Lycopodium, Nux vomica
Aching	Gelsemium
Acidity	Lycopodium
Air sickness	Belladonna
Alcohol	Ignatia, Kali bich., Nux vomica
Allergic reaction	Apis
Anesthetic	Calendula, Hypericum
Angriness	Pulsatilla, Sepia
Antibiotic	Echinacea
Antiseptic	Calendula, Hypericum
Anxiety	Aconite, Arsenicum, Gelsemium
Arthritis	Kali bich.
Asthma	Aconite, Nux vomica
Attention	Chamomilla
Bee sting	Apis, Arnica
Belching	Cantharis
Bites	Ledum
Bladder	Cantharis, Staphasagria, Pulsatilla
Blister	Cantharis
Bloating	Lycopodium
Blow	Hypericum
Boils	Belladonna, Hepar sulph., Ferrum phos.
Bronchitis	Bryonia, Ipecac
Bruising	Arnica, Ledum
Burn	Cantharis
Carbuncle	Arsenicum
Cat bite	Hypericum
Catarrh	Arsenicum, Kali bich.
Chickenpox	Belladonna, Rhus tox.
Chilly	Hepar sulph.
Coccyx	Hypericum
Coffee	Calc. carb., Ignatia, Nux vomica
Colds	Aconite, Belladonna, Bryonia, Calc. carb., Dulcamara, Echinacea, Ferrum phos., Gelsemium
Cold sore	Rhus tox.
Colic	Aethusa

SYMPTOMS	REMEDIES
Conjunctivitis	Pulsatilla
Cough	Aconite, Bryonia, Hepar sulph., Rhus tox.
Day care illness	Echinacea
Dental	Arnica
Depression	Ignatia
Diaper rash	Calendula
Diarrhea	Arsenicum, Bryonia
Disrespect	Staphasagria
Dizziness	Gelsemium
Draft	Calc. carb., Hepar sulph.
Dryness	Bryonia
Ear	Belladonna, Hepar sulph.
Eczema	Calendula, Rhus tox.
Edema	Apis
Egg cravings	Calc. carb.
Emphysema	Carbo. veg.
Exams	Gelsemium
Eye	Dulcamara, Euphrasia, Gelsemium
Eyelid	Apis, Pulsatilla
Face	Ferrum phos.
Failure	Lycopodium
Fainting	Sepia
Falls	Hypericum
Fatty food	Nux vomica, Pulsatilla
Fear	Aconite, Arsenicum, Ignatia
Feet	Calc. carb.
Fever	Bryonia
Finger	Hypericum
Fish	Carbo. veg.
Fishbone	Hepar sulph.
Floating	Hypericum
Flu	Aconite, Dulcamara, Echinacea, Gelsemium
Flush	Belladonna, Gelsemium
Forehead	Gelsemium
Fretfulness	Chamomilla
Fruit (too much)	Arsenicum, Bryonia

SYMPTOMS	REMEDIES
Frustration	Ignatia
Fussiness	Chamomilla
Gas	Cantharis, Carbo. veg., Lycopodium
Gout	Arnica, Bryonia
Grief	Aconite, Ignatia
Gums	Apis
Hand	Calc. carb.
Hangover	Nux vomica
Hay fever	Arsenicum, Pulsatilla
Headache	Belladonna, Chamomilla, Ferrum phos., Gelsemium, Ignatia, Kali bich., Thuja
Heartburn	Carbo. veg., Lycopodium, Nux vomica
Hernia	Lycopodium, Nux vomica
Hiccough	Lycopodium
Hip	Bryonia
Hives	Apis
Hormones	Sepia
Hot weather	Kali bich.
Humidity	Pulsatilla
Hunger	Lycopodium
Hypertension	Carbo. veg.
Hysteria	Ignatia
Immunization	Thuja
Impatience	Chamomilla
Incontinence	Apis, Belladonna, Sepia
Indigestion	Lycopodium
Infection	Belladonna, Echinacea
Intercourse	Staphasagria
Irritability	Chamomilla, Lycopodium, Sepia
Irritation	Cantharis
Joint	Belladonna, Pulsatilla, Rhus tox.
Kidney	Apis
Knee	Bryonia

Symptoms	Remedies
Left side	Hypericum
Ligament	Rhus tox.
Lip	Bryonia
Loneliness	Bryonia
Measles	Belladonna
Meat (overeating)	Arsenicum
Menopausal flush	Belladonna, Sepia
Menopause	Pulsatilla
Migraine	Kali bich.
Milk sensitivity	Aethusa, Calc. carb.
Morning sickness	Nux vomica
Motion sickness	Ipecac, Nux vomica
Mumps	Belladonna, Pulsatilla
Muscles	Gelsemium
Mucus	Pulsatilla
Nasal discharge	Dulcamara
Nausea	Ipecac, Pulsatilla
Neck	Aconite, Belladonna, Bryonia, Gelsemium, Lycopodium, Nux vomica, Rhus tox.
Needle puncture	Ledum
Nerve	Hypericum
Nettle rash	Apis
Neuralgia	Belladonna, Gelsemium
Noise	Belladonna, Nux vomica
Nose	Dulcamara, Gelsemium
Nosebleed	Ferrum phos.
Ovarian cyst	Apis
Over-eating	Nux vomica
Over-exertion	Rhus tox.
Pain	Aconite, Apis, Arnica, Arsenicum, Bryonia, Cantharis, Chamomilla, Hypericum, Ignatia
Periods	Belladonna, Calc. carb., Chamomilla, Lycopodium, Pulsatilla, Sepia

SYMPTOMS	REMEDIES
Piles	Nux vomica
Poisoning	Carbo. veg.
Poison ivy	Rhus tox.
Rash	Calendula, Rhus tox.
Psoriasis	Arsenicum
Restlessness	Aconite, Arsenicum, Rhus tox.
Rheumatism	Bryonia, Rhus tox.
Right side	Apis
Rupture	Belladonna
Sadness	Sepia
Salt (too much)	Calc. carb.
Scald	Cantharis
Sciatica	Ignatia, Rhus tox.
Shingles	Apis
Shock	Arnica, Carbo. veg., Ignatia
Sinusitis	Hepar sulph., Kali bich., Pulsatilla
Skin	Calc. carb., Hepar sulph.
Sleeplessness	Arnica, Nux vomica, Thuja
Sneezing	Gelsemium
Spinal anesthetic	Ledum
Spine	Hypericum
Sprain	Arnica, Rhus tox.
Splinter	Hypericum, Ledum
Stomach	Arsenicum, Bryonia
Sunburn	Cantharis
Sunstroke	Belladonna, Gelsemium
Surgery	Arnica, Rhus tox.
Swallowing	Gelsemium
Sweat	Calc. carb., Hepar sulph., Sepia, Thuja
Sweets (too many)	Calc. carb., Ignatia, Lycopodium
Synovitis	Apis
Teething	Aconite, Apis, Belladonna, Chamomilla
Tendon	Rhus tox.
Thirst	Bryonia, Pulsatilla, Rhus tox.
Throat	Aconite, Apis, Arsenicum
Tinnitus	Aconite, Lycopodium
Tobacco	Aconite, Calc. carb., Ignatia, Nux vomica, Sepia

Symptoms	Remedies
Toes	Hypericum
Tonsillitis	Aconite, Apis, Belladonna, Hypericum, Lycopodium
Toothache	Aconite, Arnica, Belladonna
Tongue	Bryonia
Travel sickness	Nux vomica
Ulcer	Belladona, Carbo. veg., Sepia
Urine	Cantharis, Lycopodium, Thuja, Nux vomica
Varicose veins	Carbo. veg.
Voice loss	Arnica, Belladonna
Vomit	Arsenicum, Ferrum phos., Ipecac
Vulnerability	Staphasagria, Nux vomica, Pulsatilla
Warts	Calc. carb., Sepia, Thuja
Weight	Calc. carb.
Whining	Chamomilla
Wind	Carbo. veg.
Wine	Calc. carb.
Worry	Ignatia, Rhus box.
Wound	Calendula, Hypericum

RESOURCES

Candida Research and Information Foundation
P.O. Box 2719
Castro Valley, CA 94546

Homeopathic remedies and remedy kits may be obtained from your homeopathic physician, your local health food store, or by mail order from:
Homeopathic Educational Services
2124 Kittredge St.
Berkeley, CA 94704
(800) 359-9051

REFERENCE BOOKS

Childhood Ear Infections by Michael Schmidt, D.C.
Creative Visualization by Shakti Gawain
Cross Currents by Robert O. Becker, M.D.
Diet For a New America by John Robbins
Dr. Atkins' Health Revolution by Robert C. Atkins, M.D.
Eating Alive by John Madden, N.D.
Fast Food Guide by Michael F. Jacobson, Ph.D. and Sarah Fritschner
Fats and Oils by Udo Erasmus
Feed Your Kids Right by Lendon Smith, M.D.

Healing With Nutrition by Jonathan Wright, M.D.

Herbally Yours by Penny C. Royal

Homeopathy: Medicine for the 21st Century by Dana Ullman

The Hug Therapy Book by Kathleen Keating

Hypothyroidism; The Unsuspected Illness by Broda O. Barnes, M.D.

The Missing Diagnosis by Orian Truss, M.D.

No Immediate Danger: Prognosis for a Radioactive Earth by Rosalie
Bertell, Ph.D.

Nutraerobics by Jeffrey Bland, Ph.D.

Peak Immunity by Luc De Schepper, M.D.

The Relaxation Response by Herbert Benson, M.D.

Take Charge of Your Body by Carolyn DeMarco, M.D.

Understanding Menopause by Janine O'Leary Cobb

Why Your House May Endanger Your Health by Alfred Zamm, M.D.
and Robert Gannon

A Woman's Guide to Homeopathic Medicine by Trevor Smith, M.D.

The Yeast Connection by William Crook, M.D.

The Yeast Syndrome by John P. Trowbridge, M.D. and Morton
Walker, D.P.M.

You Don't Have to Live with Cystitis by Larrian Gillespie, M.D.

Your Body's Many Cries for Water by F. Batmanghelidj, M.D.

Your Health Under Seige by Jeffrey Bland, Ph.D.

INDEX

abdominal pain, 178
aching, 178
acid balance of body and psoriasis, 138
acidity, 178
acidophilus, how to take, 2, 3
  for Candidiasis, 47–48; in babies, 25
  for canker sores, 50
  for diabetes, 67
  for diarrhea, 68
  for gas, 91
  for travel diarrhea, 149
  for vaginitis, 152
acne, 1–3
Aconite (homeopathic), 156–157
  for agoraphobia, 7
  for asthma, 19
  for childbirth, 134
  for colds and flu, 56
  for earaches, 76
  for fever in babies, 26
acupuncture
  for asthma, 19
  for bursitis, 44
  for endometriosis, 80
  for smoking, 4
addictions, 3–6
adrenal supplement
  for hypoglycemia, 107
  for menopause, 120

Aethusa (homeopathic), 157
  for colic in babies, 58
agoraphobia, 6–7
air sickness, 178
alcohol addiction, 5–6, 178
alfalfa tablets for psoriasis, 138
allergic headaches, 97
allergies
  and asthma, 18–19
  and diabetes, 66
  babies and, 21–22
  challenge test for food allergies, 8
  inhalant, 9
aloe vera gel
  acne treatment, 2
  for arteriosclerosis, 16
  for detoxification, 65
  for headaches, 97
  for sunburn, 146
  for ulcers, 152
  for warts, 154
alum for canker sores, 50
Alumina (homeopathic) for constipation, 62
aluminum antacids and constipation, 61
Ambrosia (homeopathic ragweed) for allergies, 7
amenorrhea (absence of menstruation), 9–10